PUSH-UP
PROGRESSION

A 24 PUSH-UP JOURNEY TO STABILIZATION, STRENGTH, AND POWER

**2ND
EDITION**

Published by Price World Publishing
3971 Hoover Rd. Suite 77
Columbus, OH 43123-2839

Book Interior Design by Merwin Loquias
Cover Design by Russell Marleau
Editing by Vanessa Fravel
Photographs by Rebecca Weiss Photography
Printing by Cushing-Malloy, Inc.

First Edition, 2012
ISBN: 9781932549850
eISBN: 9781619843615
LCCN: 2014952170

Printed in the United States of America
10 9 8 7 6 5 4 3 2 1

PUSH-UP
PROGRESSION

A 24 PUSH-UP JOURNEY TO STABILIZATION, STRENGTH, AND POWER

2ND EDITION

PRICE WORLD
PUBLISHING

In dedication to my sweet fiancée Adrienne, my loving family, supportive friends, loyal clientele, and all of the fitness professionals who inspire me.

Table of Contents

INTRODUCTION

This book speaks to the benefit of progression and executing the otherwise "traditional push-up" by performing a series of eight push-ups via stabilization, strength, and power techniques for a total of 24 push-ups that will challenge you unlike any other push-up you have performed before. This book discusses how instrumental the push-up is in regards to training the core, upper body, and lower body.

Everyone can benefit from reading this book because this program provides: core stabilization, improved posture, increased power, extra endurance, stronger stability in your joints, more strength in their upper and lower body, increased muscle mass, and fat loss.

While you discover how to improve your push-up technique, a main goal of this book is to inspire you to appreciate the benefits of refining your push-up approach in meeting your overall fitness training goals. You will not only become more advanced at performing the push-up with proper form, but you will also gain optimal core stabilization and core movement muscles that will functionally improve your posture. Obtaining optimal posture is vital for anyone to create proper symmetry via muscle length tension relationships in the body.

Mastering the push-up is important because while some individuals can press heavy weights at the gym, their actual true strength may not compare when it comes to performing the push-ups in this book. Push-ups challenge your core stability and core movement muscles more so than most exercises you might perform in a typical workout routine. Similarly, both the beginner and professional alike may be unaware of the extensive values that push-ups provide in conditioning the entire body.

Beyond the common desire to have stronger arms and shoulders, most individuals need to improve their core stabilization muscles because you need optimal stability before you can move efficiently. Furthermore, core movement muscles are engaged during all movement and, therefore, these muscle need to be developed to execute optimal strength. The different levels of progression in this book will work your overall stability, strength, and power without using any equipment in the process. All you need to perform these push-ups is your own body and the will to continue on this push-up journey.

This journey includes various sections in which you will learn about the core stabilization and core movement muscles with their importance in gaining overall stability, strength, and power. Moreover, this book will help you identify your own over-active (tight) and under-active (weak) muscles and how these specific muscles either help or hinder in your daily life. Whereas being able to execute a proper push-up is one thing, understanding its true power and function within in your body is another complete concept.

Simply put, the push-up is an incredible exercise that offers a multitude of gains that should be implemented in your current workout routine no matter your current fitness level. In essence, if you are able to execute a variety of push-ups, with the aforementioned goals in mind, the benefits of this program are plentiful. Whether you're someone who can devote hours weekly to this program or a very busy person with a limited schedule, performing a few exercises in this book, even on occasion, would be valuable. Therefore, this book can benefit anyone and everyone no matter your fitness goals, levels, and lifestyle.

PART 1

Core

The core remains a very popular word these days in the world of fitness. Most of us have seen or heard this term used frequently in magazines, TV commercials, or online articles, at your local gym, or even from your friends. While most of us know that having a strong core is fundamental, let's take a more detailed look into why a stronger core is crucially beneficial for everyone.

What is the Core?

The core can be best characterized as the central area of the body that consists of your entire spine (cervical, thoracic, and lumbar), the pelvic girdle, and hip flexors. Your core encompasses all of the core stabilization and core movement muscles that include your abdominals and obliques. Your core goes beyond just your abdominal muscles since your other core muscles are the gluteus maximus, gluteus medius, gluteus minimus, anterior shoulders, medial shoulders, posterior shoulders, pectoralis major muscles, pectoralis minor muscles, latissimus dorsi, and scapulae. Thus, the core consists not just of your abdominals or lower back, but includes a multitude of muscles, tendons, bones, and joints. Essentially, the core can be defined as your entire body excluding the extremities such as your head, arms, and legs.

Anatomy of the Core

These muscles of the core can be classified into distinct categories based upon their function of either stabilizing or providing movement for your body.

The core stabilization muscles are:

- ▶ Transverse Abdominis
- ▶ Internal Oblique
- ▶ Pelvic Floor
- ▶ Multifidus
- ▶ Diaphragm
- ▶ Transversospinalis

The core movement muscles are:

▸ Rectus Abdominis
▸ External Oblique
▸ Latissimus Dorsi
▸ Erector Spinae
▸ Iliopsoas
▸ Hip Adductors
▸ Hip Abductors

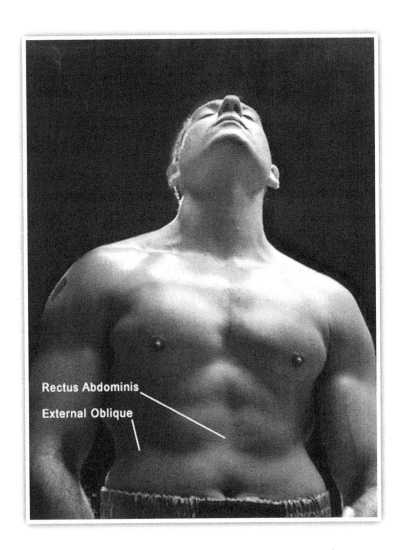

Rectus Abdominis

External Oblique

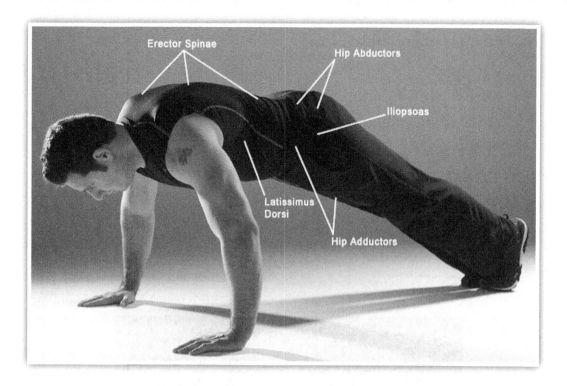

All of the core muscles in these two categories must work together as one functional unit in order to provide optimal stabilization and movement of the body. These muscles must be trained correctly for optimal functional activity, or compensations most likely will occur from inefficient movements. Performing inefficient movements consistently over time can lead to opportunities for the body to become injured. Therefore, it's vital to train these muscles for core stabilization first. Then, once these core muscles have become stable, the next step would be to train the core muscles that provide movement. For example, when starting a core training routine, you'd always want to functionally perform a plank first because the plank incorporates most of the core stabilization muscles and even more stability in your hip flexors. After your core stabilization muscles are strong from the plank, then you could attempt to perform other core movement exercises such as a crunch. Crunches engage the core movement muscles, however, they do not engage your entire rectus abdominis, and they tighten your hip flexors and psoas major muscles. A better choice for an abdominal exercise to engage the rectus abdominis would be a lying leg raise. *Regardless of your choice of core movement exercise, the formula for a stronger core should always be training the core stabilization muscles first and then the core movement muscles secondarily.* Therefore, the 24 push-ups in this book include the core stabilization push-ups *first* that teach you how to engage your optimal core stabilization muscles. Then as you continue your push-up journey, more advanced push-ups in this book include a variety of the core movement muscles via strength and power.

Functions of the Core

Core Stabilization Muscles

Transverse Abdominis

The transverse abdominis is the innermost abdominal muscle in your body. The transverse abdominis is the only abdominal muscle to attach to the posterior spine. It acts as an internal "weight belt" and supplies thoracic and pelvic stability to your vertebral column. A stable spine is imperative in order to properly perform movements and exercises with optimal function. The transverse abdominis keeps your abdominals aesthetically "flat" and engaged.

Internal Oblique

The internal oblique is positioned underneath the external oblique. This muscle helps stabilize the inner abdominals, assists an involuntary breathing, helps in raising the inner abdominal compression, and rotates and abducts the abdominals with help from other muscles. Internal abdominal oblique muscles are often referred to as side rotators. Both sides of your oblique muscles function together when providing flexion and rotation to the abdominals.

Pelvic Floor

The pelvic floor consists of multiple muscles that are superficial and multi-layered.

Pelvic floor muscles provide two major functions for your body. First, they create a "floor" to your abdominal viscera. Second, a strong pelvic floor assists in helping both men and women who have problems with urine seepage and/or bowel control.

Multifidus

The multifidus is one of the smallest abdominal muscles, yet is crucial because it performs assistance to spinal stability. The areas of the spine that contain your multifidus include the sacral, lumbar, thoracic, and cervical. This muscle permits your spine to remain straight, and therefore, perform efficient and functional activity.

Diaphragm

The diaphragm is a large, flat muscle that is usually referred to as "dome shaped." This muscle separates the chest from the abdominal muscles. The diaphragm is attached to the spine, ribs, and sternum in both the abdominal cavity and the thoracic cavity. The main function of the diaphragm is breathing and respiration.

Transversospinalis

The transversospinalis is a collection of very small muscles located in your vertebral column. These muscles include: semispinalis dorsi, semispinalis cervicis, semispinalis capitis, multifidus, rotatores, rotatores cervicis, rotatores thoracis, rotatores lumborum, interspinales, and intertransversarii. All of these muscles work together to provide extension and rotation in your body.

The core stabilization muscles in your body must function with the best possible efficiency in order to operate optimal strength, balance, endurance, and power. If these muscles are weak, this again will most likely result in injuries, most commonly developing into chronic lower back pain. Therefore, individuals who do not strength train their core stabilization muscles are more susceptible to injuries than those who don't. The first section of your push-up journey focuses on optimizing these stabilization muscles. This will be the foundation from which you will then be able to move efficiently with strength and power.

Core Movement Muscles

Rectus Abdominis

The rectus abdominis is possibly the most commonly known core movement muscle since it comprises the ever-popular "six-pack." This long abdominal muscle extends vertically the full length of your anterior torso. The main function of the rectus abdominis is to create flexion to the lumbar vertebrae while also creating flexion of the ribs while bringing your pelvis inward.

External Oblique

The external oblique is one of the largest core movement muscles. It is one of the most superficial layers extending all the way upward towards your chest muscles. The external oblique has many functions that include: helping with full rotation of your abdominals, providing assistance while drawing your chest downward from abdominal compression, and delivering assistance in rotation of the spine.

Latissimus Dorsi

The latissimus dorsi is both the widest and largest muscle in your back. Moreover, it's the only muscle in your upper body that connects to your lower body. The main functions of this muscle are: creating extension, adduction, horizontal abduction, and rotation to your shoulders and arms. As it pertains to the core movement muscles, your latissimus dorsi provides flexion to your spine.

Erector Spinae

The erector spinae are a series of muscles and tendons that run vertically through the lumbar, thoracic, and cervical regions of your spine. The assembly of muscles that make up your erector spinae aid in extending, bending, and twisting your spine in a variety of directions, in addition to providing spinal stability while standing.

Iliopsoas

Your iliopsoas consists of your psoas muscle and iliacus. The main function of your iliopsoas is to generate flexion to your hips. If your iliopsoas is over-active (tight) then this could lead to muscular imbalances such as an anterior pelvic tilt. However, the iliopsoas can facilitate movement in your abdominals by creating flexion and rotation to your spine.

Hip Adductors

The hip adductors consists of a series of muscles that include: adductor brevis, adductor longus, adductor magnus, adductor minimus, pectineus, gracilis, and the obturator externus. The main function of the hip adductors is to adduct (move the leg towards) the hip joint. Additionally, other functions of these adductor muscles are transverse adduction, internal and external rotation, and extension for the hips. As a result, these core movement muscles play a vital role to your abdominals.

Hip Abductors

The hip abductors are a group of muscles that consist of: gluteus minimus, gluteus medius, tensor fasciae latae, piriformis, and sartorius. It's worth noting that the sartorius is the longest muscle in your body. The main function of the hip abductor muscles is to abduct (move the leg away from) the hip joint. These muscles also provide stabilization to your pelvis either while moving or standing.

The core can be considered the first muscles that become engaged with movement. They are the center of gravity to the body. If the core movement muscles are inadequate, they cannot provide proper assistance to the core stabilization muscles. The bottom line is: *when the core stabilization and core movement muscles are working at optimal levels, you will activate the proper muscles necessary for stability and movement. In addition, you will obtain more overall muscle engagement within your entire body, including supporting weak muscles that may otherwise hinder your ability to execute a movement efficiently.* For example, if an individual is attempting a traditional push-up and has very strong core stabilization muscles, but lacks strength in their upper body, their core stabilization muscles will help facilitate the upper body muscles to become stronger when performing the push-up. This cycle can even apply to your weight training, as developing a stronger core from push-ups will assist with pressing more weight at the gym. In fact, performing the push-ups in this book will produce more overall stability, strength, and power with any exercise you perform.

Posture

Since the core can be defined as the entire spine, having optimal stabilization and movement in your core muscles is critical for the best possible posture. However, as mentioned above, when training the core for optimal posture, everyone must strength train their core stabilization muscles first and core movement muscles second.

Many of us struggle with trying to obtain good posture. In fact, millions of Americans suffer from lower back pain, which can be prevented by having stronger core stabilization and core movement muscles. Poor posture can lead to an incredible amount of muscular imbalances and compensations in your body. Therefore, those with poor posture should be mindful of potential injury-inducing exercises and certain daily life activities. (Also, not to mention, but poor posture can be aesthetically unpleasing, too.)

Multiple activities can contribute to suboptimal posture. Namely, sitting excessively, which so many lifestyles and professions require, wreaks havoc on your posture. Furthermore, if you sit constantly for work and then travel home to spend most of your evening sitting again via watching television or eating dinner, you compound the negative effects on your spine. To troubleshoot, aim to sit no more than one to two hours at a time. Be sure to take intermittent breaks by standing up out of your seat and walk around, even if only for a brief amount of time.

Remember to do your best to always be aware of and practice proper posture while you sit, walk, or perform any other daily activity, to help assist in achieving efficient stability and mobility. Most of us are unaware of our posture and this only leads to improper habits. These bad habits will only create inefficient muscle memory to our bodies.

Performing efficient movements with optimal posture resets your muscle memory to not practice these incorrect behaviors. As stated above, the push-ups listed in this book will increase strength to your core stabilization and core movement muscles to help functionally create optimal posture.

If you suffer from any postural disorders, then please skip to the Muscular Imbalance section of this book before performing any of the push-ups listed. Also, please also reference the stretching section of this book for proper guidance on over-active (tight) muscles.

Drawing-In Maneuver

When strength training the core stabilization and core movement muscles it is ideal to "draw in" your abdominals right before performing a core exercise. To perform correctly, "suck" in your abdominals towards the spine. This maneuver keeps constant engagement of your core stabilization and core movement muscles. This maneuver also creates better stabilization for the pelvis and therefore, more overall strength in your core. Moreover, drawing-in your abdominals helps aids your spine in finding the neutral spinal position, the common starting point of any correct push-up. Be sure to properly breathe out of your mouth and nose while performing the drawing-in maneuver for proper efficiency. Note that by also maintaining a neutral spinal position during push-ups, you will develop improved posture, muscle balance, and overall stabilization.

PART II

Push-ups

What is a Push-up?

Push-ups are an anaerobic body-weight exercise performed in the prone (chest down) position on the transverse plane (horizontal plane) by flexing the elbows at 90-degrees while the arms are used to help lower and raise the body. The gravity and resistance that the body provides during this exercise create functional and overall strength. Functional strength can best be defined as exercising to become stronger to assist in the performance of daily activities. This strength produces more stabilization and better movement of the body.

Push-ups can be considered a "moveable plank" since the core is utilized for strength just as much as the upper body is during execution. Correct push-ups should be performed with the upper body, torso, and lower body moving as one unit. Push-ups are a tremendous exercise because of the multi-joint and multiple muscle groups recruited during movement. Moreover, and most importantly, push-ups are a true test of stability, strength, and power. Push-ups also help increase endurance as a result of the volume performed in a workout. Not to mention, push-ups can be performed almost anywhere without the need of joining a gym or leaving the comfort of your own home.

The push-up and the core should work together in perfect harmony for optimal push-up performance. When mastered, the push-up with optimal core stabilization and core movement becomes the ideal training exercise because it supports many different forms of physical training. To explain, if you have a weak core, but strong upper body pressing ability, attempting a traditional push-up at first might prove challenging when trying to utilize core stability and strength. It might also be difficult to find or keep a neutral spinal position while performing the push-up. However, if you properly engage the correct core muscles during every push-up exercise featured in this book, eventually the core stabilization and core movement muscles will become stronger. Inherently, the rest of your body will become stronger, too!

While the push-up is considered one of the most popular exercises in the world, many still perform them with incorrect form and do not properly engage the right muscles for strength, stabilization, and power. Furthermore, with so many push-up variations out there, some including the support of inanimate objects, it can prove difficult to perform the seemingly simple push-up with optimal efficiency. With proper posture, form, and core engagement, this book will show you how you can more quickly see physical results of every push-up you execute, with improved musculature in other areas you may not have expected!

Benefits of Push-ups

Push-ups are considered a strength training exercise, although, the push-ups in this book promote cardiovascular health, too. Strength training provides hypertrophy, weight loss, stronger bones, and even gives you more energy! Hypertrophy is the act of increasing muscle. Unfortunately, as we all grow older, we lose muscle and even the ability for muscle to function properly via stability and mobility. This condition is called sarcopenia. Furthermore, what's extremely alarming and quite scary, is that those who chose a sedentary lifestyle lose anywhere from three to five percent of muscle every ten years starting at the age of 30! Regardless, even if you happen to live an active lifestyle, you will still acquire minor forms of sarcopenia with age. You can certainly minimize the effects of sarcopenia by maintaining an active lifestyle, and ingesting adequate amounts of protein for optimal muscle repair. Muscle is increased in your body by performing consistent exercise programs that challenge the volume of sets, repetitions, and tempo during execution. Moreover, including different plane of motions while exercising your arms and legs at various angles is essential for obtaining more muscle. While building more muscle is ideal, every time you exercise, your body changes your metabolism for the better. As a result, a faster metabolism accounts for aiding increased fat loss!

Additionally, strength training helps prevent heart disease, diabetes, cancer, stroke, hypertension, obesity, and arthritis. Consequently, those who live an inactive lifestyle and don't move on a regular basis can be at risk for a heart attack or other life-threatening diseases. Let's be clear, living a sedentary lifestyle only promotes unhealthy practices, which limits your body into achieving optimal performance. Cardiovascular exercises produce improved oxygen flow in your body and potentially decrease the probability of congestive heart failure.

Performing push-ups with increased volume (sets and repetitions) and the power push-ups in this book will provide cardiovascular exercise to fortify your cardiovascular system and your heart.

There are many other incredible benefits that exercising and performing the push-ups in this book provide. Exercising is proven to relieve stress, chronic anxiety, and depression. While working out and performing push-ups, your body produces an increased amount of the brain chemical serotonin. If serotonin levels are low, depression can occur. Strength training can also prevent cognitive brain decline in conditions such as Parkinson's disease and Alzheimer's dementia. Did you know that exercising improves brain function and sharpens your memory? That's because exercising triggers vast production of neurons, which control nervous system functions, including muscle engagement and movement. Exercising also promotes production of endorphins. Endorphins are the brain chemical that creates the sensation of happiness. Remember, if your mind is feeling stress then your body suffers, too. Performing these push-ups can certainly provide relief from stress to your mind and body (which is particularly beneficial for individuals prone to anxiety). Going forward, this exercise program can increase your self-esteem and confidence levels from a biological level even before you see the physical results. As such, think of how these outcomes can influence every endeavor you take on in your professional and personal life!

Moving on, push-ups are an incredible exercise for the amount of muscle groups that become engaged when executed. Push-ups build lean muscle in your anterior, medial, and posterior deltoid muscles, pectoralis major and pectoralis minor muscles, and triceps. Additionally, certain push-ups listed in this book engage your upper trapezius, middle trapezius, lower trapezius, rhomboids, latissimus dorsi, rotator cuffs, serratus anterior, hip flexors, erector spinae, gluteus maximus, gluteus minimus muscles, gluteus medius, quadriceps, hamstrings, and calves.

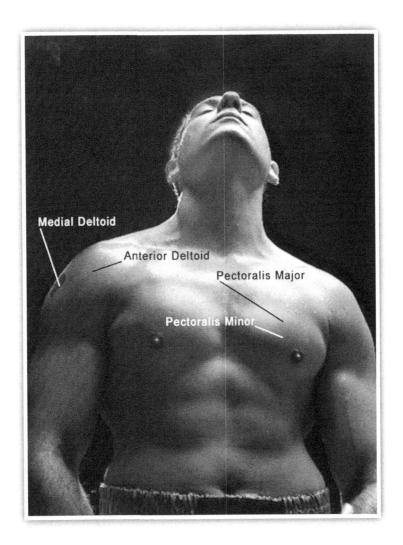

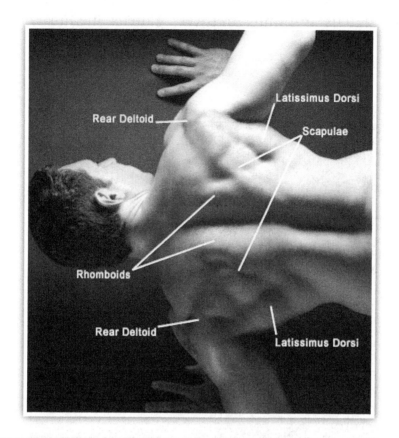

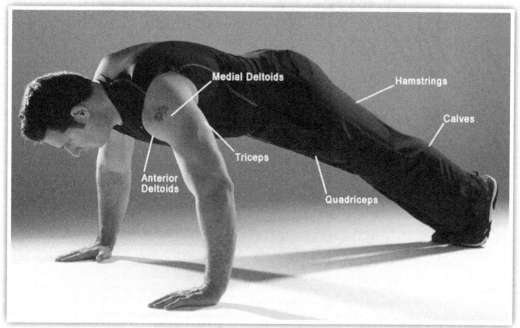

The Stabilization Push-ups section in this book engages the following core muscles: transverse abdominis, internal oblique, pelvic floor, multifidus, diaphragm, and transversospinalis. While the Strength Push-ups and Power Push-ups sections in this book engage the core stabilization muscles, their primary function is to engage the core movement muscles, which are: rectus abdominis, external oblique, latissimus dorsi, erector spinae, iliopsoas, hip adductors, and hip abductors.

The push-ups in this book will benefit everyone and anyone no matter what your fitness level. Furthermore, no matter what your fitness goals are, from building more lean muscle, creating more weight loss, or functionally becoming stronger, this program will help you achieve all of these goals.

If you don't have the time to travel to a gym or even an hour to exercise at home, performing even 10 to 15 minutes of these push-ups will yield the awesome effects of the mental and physical benefits of exercise. All of these valuable neurological and physical advantages of working out are just another reminder that making the commitment and finding the time to exercise are so important. So enjoy the push-ups in this book while you experience the euphoria!

Neutral Spinal Position

The neutral spinal position can best be defined when the top of your shoulders, middle of your back, and gluteus maximus muscles are all perfectly aligned. This position must always be maintained during every push-up for correct core and muscle engagement. The neutral spinal position supports efficient movements for the body and even helps develop optimal posture post-exercise. It's important to note that drawing in the abdominals towards your spine and engaging your gluteal muscles also supports in creating more overall stability to perform the neutral spinal position. Finally, and most importantly, this positioning in your spine encourages more overall strength for your body when performing exercises such as push-ups.

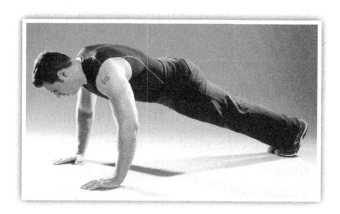

Be aware that it can be difficult to maintain the neutral spinal position during certain push-ups featured in this book. Therefore, remember to be incredibly cautious not to have your lower back form an inward curve, causing your hips to drop excessively. Similarly, do not round your upper back, which only enables the scapulae muscles to retract. Scapulae retraction is an inefficient function of the scapulae muscles since this positioning leads to loss of optimal strength, diminished range of motion, and poor posture. Moreover, scapulae retraction in this pronated position raises your gluteus maximus muscles higher than your hips. All of these incorrect methods can cause stress to your lower back, jeopardizing development of functional core strength in the core stabilization and core movement muscles.

Tips on Finding the Neutral Spinal Position

Depending on your fitness levels, attempting to find and maintain the neutral spinal position during your push-up workout can prove overwhelming. After all, you will be navigating this journey by innate skill, muscle memory, and sensation while performing the various push-ups in this book. Remember, never to forget the importance of keeping the neutral spinal position throughout. As stated above, performing the neutral spinal position is critical to avoid possible injury. It might be challenging to know where your hips and lower back are positioned since you are looking downward while in the pronated position (with your chest facing the floor). The following section provides three essential tips to develop the neutral spinal position.

If you happen to have a muscular imbalance issue such as an anterior pelvic tilt, then please skip to the Muscular Imbalance section in this book, before beginning your push-up journey.

Perform the traditional push-up position as if executing a push-up while finding your neutral spinal position. Then, have a friend or family member take a picture of you and review the image to study your form. This picture can serve two purposes. First, it can aid as a useful device in helping you remember what your body should look like in this correct spinal position. Second, the act of "finding" the correct position can actually help your muscles "remember" how to find and maintain this position more efficiently. Your muscles do have a memory, and creating muscle memory is beneficial to your body while exercising, especially in the pronated position. Be sure to study the picture and refine your posture until perfect, even if multiple trials and pictures are necessary, until you obtain that perfect shape.

Remember, it is crucial that you master the neutral spinal position before starting your push-up journey.

Mirror

The mirror can be a great instrument to help find and re-find the neutral spinal position as you execute the push-ups in this book, especially if you are still unsure of how it should feel or look. Position a mirror where you can view your entire spine while exercising. Use the mirror as often as needed to confirm the neutral spinal position until you are confident that you have mastered this positioning *without* needing to check your form visually. Just remember to avoid looking in the mirror while actually executing the push-ups, since turning your head and spine to one side mid-motion could strain your neck and/or upper trapezius muscles.

Mat

A mat can be a wonderful guide to aide in hand positioning, acting as another visual tool in achieving the neutral spinal position. Proper hand placement is key before executing any push-up to ensure correct alignment; otherwise, the neutral spinal position will not be achieved. For example, most of the non-staggered push-ups listed in this book have your hands positioned slightly wider than shoulder-width apart. Hence, a mat can serve as the helpful visual guide in placing your hands at the edge of the mat or just outside the mat (depending on the width of your shoulders).

Hand Positioning and Elbow Movement

Hand positioning and elbow movement are crucial in placement when executing a push-up for a variety of reasons. Foremost, placing your hands incorrectly can cause unnecessary strain to your muscles and even your joints. This could result in muscle compensations by creating inefficient movements and therefore injuries. In addition, because hand positioning can be so subtle during a push-up, performing the correct form is also critical to engage the exact muscles to build muscle hypertrophy and to naturally engage the correct core stabilization and movement muscles.

With *most* non-staggered hand positions in this book, your hands should be placed a little more than shoulder-width apart, aligned with your pectoralis major muscles (chest muscles). This is the correct hand positioning to build lean muscle in your chest and to distribute proper hypertrophy in your shoulders, triceps, and back muscles. For example, if your hands are positioned farther away from your torso and not aligned with your chest muscles, the push-up would distribute more lean muscle to your anterior deltoids (shoulders) instead of incorporating your chest muscles. Moreover, this hand positioning over time could cause severe injury to your shoulders, since this movement would be incredibly stressful on your shoulders if performed on a constant basis.

Again, hand placement does matter in terms of which muscles you'd want to properly engage. Creating internal rotation in your hands positioning (when your hands rotate inward) is not correct form. This form could result in injury because it once again puts unwanted strain on your shoulders, rotator cuffs, and your wrists. Also, if your hands are naturally rotated inward, then your anterior shoulders are most likely over-active (tight) and need to be properly stretched.

It's crucial to keep in the mind that engaging a muscle via strength training over time will tighten (shorten) this muscle. As a result, performing the push-ups in this book will tighten your chest and shoulder muscles, thus, you might see your wrists wanting naturally to internally rotate. This is your body's method of explaining that certain muscles in the anterior chain (chest, shoulders, and triceps) are over-active (tight) and need to be properly stretched. Don't be alarmed though, this book provides the correct stretches to correct this issue if needed.

Next, elbow movement during push-up execution is equally as important. Elbow inflammation and strains are quite common in the world of fitness due to repetitive movements or performing an exercise incorrectly over time. Performing a push-up correctly absolutely depends on what direction your elbow is bending (flexing). While performing a traditional push-up your elbows should be descending downward into a 90-degree angle to recruit a proper balance of chest, shoulder, and triceps muscle recruitment. In contrast, during the "staggered" push-ups in this book, your front elbow should be bent downward into a 90-degree angle, while your rear elbow should be bent at 40-degree angle to recruit the proper chest, shoulder, and triceps muscle recruitment.

Whether you are performing the Traditional Push-up, Staggered Push-up, or Jumping Jack Push-up in this book, do not create more than a 90-degree angle while bending your elbows since this repetitive flexion in your elbow could yield injury to your shoulders, elbow tendon, and wrist joints. Moreover, with either of these push-ups, do not let your elbows flair out to the side past your wrists. This kind of elbow flexion puts an incredible strain on your elbow joints and will not engage the proper chest, shoulder, and triceps muscles to build hypertrophy. Performing the correct hand positioning and elbow movement will build the proper muscle in your body, creating the correct functional strength that push-ups require, while keeping you safe from potential injury.

PART III

Tips to Maximize Your Efforts

Gluteus Maximus

The gluteus maximus is integral in many functions of the body by creating movement patterns of hip flexion and hip extension, hip internal rotation and hip external rotation, and hip addiction and hip abduction. You may not realize it, but the gluteus maximus muscles can serve as a functional support system to initiate overall strength while performing a push-up, too! You have three gluteus muscles: gluteus maximus, gluteus medius, and the gluteus minimius. All three are engaged during push-ups, although the gluteus maximus obtains the highest engagement during the performance of push-ups. However, there are some specific push-up exercises in this book that target your gluteus medius and gluteus minimius. The gluteus maximus is considered the biggest muscle group in your body and also can be the strongest, too. Therefore, let's remember to always engage these gluteal muscles to assist during your push-ups.

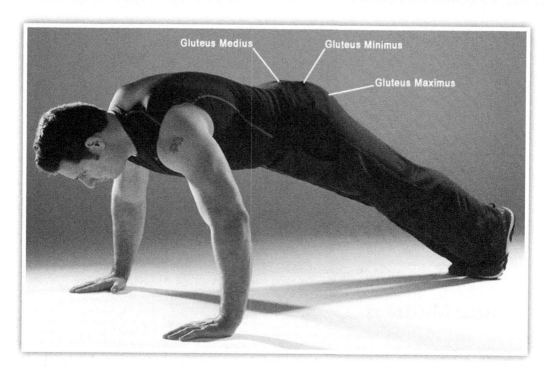

Actively engaging your gluteus maximus muscles, thereby making them stronger, helps you perform push-ups more easily, and can also help you in finding and maintaining the neutral spinal position. It's crucial that the gluteus maximus muscles are strong, because when they are weak, various compensations can occur in the body. Your gluteus maximus muscles become weak due to inactivity, which mostly stems from sitting excessively, since your hip flexors become tighter. Gluteus maximus muscles could also be considered "lazy" since every day basic activities such as sitting or even walking don't engage your gluteal muscles to their highest potential. In contrast, performing exercises such as: lunging, squatting, jumping, and naturally, push-ups, all strengthen your gluteus maximus.

Compensations from these weak gluteal muscles can lead to the over-stressing of certain muscles, which can result in strain and even injury. Specifically, muscular imbalances in the pelvis can prevent you from performing and maintaining the neutral spinal position during push-ups. For example, if you have anterior pelvic tilt (later explained in the Muscular Imbalances section) your gluteal muscles and core muscles are very weak, while your hip flexors and quadriceps are over-active (tight). Stronger gluteus maximus muscles aid in achieving optimal posture and help prevent muscular imbalances that can occur in the pelvis, which can lead to the prevention of lower back strains.

Another benefit of engaging your gluteus maximus muscles during push-ups is that lean muscle can be created along with efficient functional strength. Push-ups can provide an aesthetically pleasing look to your gluteus maximus muscle. In summary: *stronger gluteal muscles benefit you in executing push-ups more efficiently and effectively, they support in obtaining the correct spinal position, they help avoid compensations and muscular imbalances in the body, and, therefore, prevent your body from possible injury.*

Breathing

Taking proper breaths is essential for achieving the best possible strength and power while performing push-ups. To execute properly, take in a deep breath as you descend into a push-up. Next, rise up and breathe out solidly as you return to the starting position. You may want to take multiple breaths during the push-up if needed to accomplish more core engagement and overall strength. Don't be afraid to make your breaths audible to help you execute them more fully and so that you maintain consistency while executing the push-up.

"The Focused Five"

Before taking the starting position of any of the push-ups below, get into the habit of remembering and applying these five key points of focus. These tips will help in aiding you with more stability, strength, and power to perform all of these push-ups. Consider these points your mantras, and let them always be your sidekick as you continue on in your push-up journey:

- ▸ Maintain a neutral spinal position
- ▸ Do not lean or hike your hips upwards
- ▸ Engage your gluteus maximus
- ▸ "Draw in" your abdominals
- ▸ Utilize your downward inhaling / upward exhaling breath

Rather than listing these points beside every exercise below, remember to apply them at all times! They are your baseline starting blocks to your 24 Push-up Journey.

The Journey

The Ultimate Push-up Progression Workout for a Stronger Core features 24 push-ups, arranged in three separate sections of eight push-ups that progress as you continue with each section. These sections are: stabilization, strength, and power to achieve the ultimate in core and muscle performance. Additionally, each push-up within each section has its own guide to three different fitness programs to help find your appropriate fitness level. These fitness levels are: beginner, intermediate, and advanced (please see the Progression section for much more detailed information). While there are numerous push-ups from which I could have chosen, I'm confident that these 24 push-ups are the most beneficial to achieve all of these fitness levels listed above. Below is a more detailed description of why each fitness section is crucial to master, and the benefits these specific push-ups in each section can provide regardless of what your fitness goals and levels are currently.

Stabilization

As stated above, you cannot create efficient movement in any exercise until you have optimal stability. Efficient movements can best be defined as generating correct movement by properly engaging the correct muscles to move. As such, stabilization exercises are the start of your push-up journey and the "building blocks" to any proper strength and eventual power program. Stabilization push-up exercises incorporate the core stabilization muscles and some of your core movement muscles as you advanced to more challenging push-ups. The core stabilization muscles can be listed as Type 1 muscle fibers since they respond best to time-under-tension of core engagement for 10 to 20 seconds per implementation.

If you consider yourself "advanced" when it comes to fitness or even a professional athlete, everyone should start with the stabilization push-up exercises in this book because of the incredible benefits they provide. A great analogy to keep in mind is to remember that we, as human beings, had to properly sit up first before we could walk. Therefore, not only do stabilization push-ups help create strength to progress you into the next strength push-up, they can provide stability to weak muscles, preventing potential muscular compensations and even possible injuries. The proper technique of isometric holding (holding without movement) your weight for several seconds to minutes at a time is helpful to building tendon strength, especially if you have a reoccurring injury (i.e. in your rotator cuffs). It's extremely beneficial to start this program or any program with "real" strength, meaning that you aren't compensating a different muscle group to create stability that provides the correct strength. Producing "false" strength by inefficiently performing stabilization exercises serves no value and will only lead to possible injuries later, especially if you carry the bad habit into more challenging push-ups. As a result, it is extremely beneficial to execute efficient stabilization exercises since this stability you perform will only benefit you as you continue to progress with the push-ups in this book or any exercise program of your choosing.

While everyone is starting out on the same push-up journey in this book, no matter what your fitness levels are currently, there are some special populations that could find this Stabilization Push-up section very valuable. For example, if you're in the senior citizen population and are presently exercising or haven't started an exercise program, performing these stability push-up exercises will help produce better bone density, stronger tendons, and correct stability needed to move more efficiently. All of these benefits lead to more functional stability, which result in easier execution of stability (balance) and movement. Next, if you are recovering from an unfortunate injury such as a strained rotator cuff or a torn tendon in your shoulders, these stability push-up exercises are again your "building blocks" for creating the proper stabilization needed to be able to efficiently move with every day functional life and naturally with exercise.

These push-ups build lean muscle in your upper body, lower body, and of course the core, while providing an aesthetically-pleasing look that most would desire. If you're someone who has had trouble building muscle and just can't put on the lean muscle mass that you desire in your upper and even lower body, these push-ups can help assist in producing hypertrophy. On the other hand, performing these stability push-up exercises can help shed excess pounds while producing lean muscle in your total body all the while promoting that flat stomach via a stronger core.

If you're trying to lose weight and are feeling discouraged, these push-ups can burn unwanted calories all day long after you are even done exercising! The reason is because of your muscle fibers, which are made up of actin and myosin. As you perform strength training exercises such as these stability push-ups, you are physically yet safely tearing the actin and myosin muscle fibers. Your body needs to then repair these fibers that were torn from exercise, and this "repairing" happens throughout the day. In contrast, aerobic (with oxygen) activity such as cardiovascular exercises on a treadmill or elliptical can result in burning many calories, but this occurs only *while* exercising. Therefore, while performing cardiovascular exercise is absolutely beneficial, performing these push-ups is even more productive in achieving weight loss even when not exercising!

Strength

After successfully completely and conquering the Stabilization Push-ups in this book, the next section to engage the proper core movement muscles is the Strength Push-up section. When your body has mastered efficient stabilization, your strength progression can flourish.

Strength push-up exercises engage more of the core movement muscles than the core stabilization muscles because you are in motion. Strength movements provide a double functional and aesthetic hit to your core since they engage both groups of core muscles.

While everyone can benefit from performing the Strength Push-up exercises in this book, they provide exceptional benefits to some special populations. For example, if you're someone who's main fitness goal is to gain more muscle because you're a body builder or an athlete, then this section will provide increased muscle mass to your entire body. However, you don't have to be a professional body builder or world-class athlete to benefit from this strength section. Those of you who are hard-gainers and are working very hard to gain muscle mass (hypertrophy) will experience encouraging results by performing the Strength Push-ups in this book.

Creating more muscle mass and building pure strength in your body are two different concepts, although these strength push-ups can combine these two notions together. First, we know that performing these strength push-ups will build more muscle in our bodies. By performing these strength push-ups you will also become stronger due to the volume of sets and repetitions. However, if your main fitness goal is to become stronger and you aren't focused on creating hypertrophy in your body, then think of the lean muscle you are building as an extraordinary bonus. The feeling of physical strength is an incredible, empowering feeling. When you feel physically stronger, you have the confidence to move as you wish or need. This feeling of independence is very empowering. Thus, if you are someone who has rehabilitated successfully from an injury or someone who has never experienced any strength in their prior fitness routines, then these strength push-ups will definitely help yield these results. Most importantly, creating strength after obtaining proper stability will benefit all of us in our every day lives. For instance, whether you are carrying your luggage at the airport, holding your beautiful baby for long periods at a time, or even moving your furniture in your home, the strength gained from these push-ups will then help you in all of your daily activities.

One of the most desired aesthetic muscles that almost all of us try to work in our current exercise programs is the rectus abdominis. The rectus abdominis is known as the famous "six pack" that most of us seem to want desperately. These "six pack" muscles are engaged during the Strength Push-ups section in this book because of the core movement that these push-ups provide. It's an interesting concept that you definitely don't need to waste excessive hours at the gym or at home performing a variety of abdominal exercises when performing these strength push-ups will engage the rectus abdominis all while saving you precious time and energy. Along with the stabilization push-ups, performing these strength push-ups can help in assisting you lose those unwanted pounds. These push-ups will also burn unwanted calories all day long after you are even done exercising due to safely tearing of the muscle fibers, actin and myosin. Performing these strength push-up exercises can unquestionably aid in building more muscle mass in your upper body, lower body, and core movement and stabilization muscles all while helping create that "six pack."

Power

Following your successfully completed sections of Stabilization and Strength, your final journey in finishing this book is the Power Push-ups section. Power can be defined as having optimal strength and quickness to perform a movement. When your body has efficient stabilization and strength levels, power progressions are able to flourish due to the force needed to perform these power movements. Many of these push-ups require you to hop or even jump utilizing your legs, while your upper body provides the proper stabilization and strength needed for optimal form.

Power push-up exercises engage more of your core movement muscles than your core stabilization muscles because you are constantly in motion. These push-ups also engage more of your posterior chain than the other push-ups sections of this book. The posterior chain muscles consist of your gluteal muscles, hamstrings, and calves. However, much as the strength push-ups in this book, power push-ups deliver a double functional and aesthetic triumph to your core since they engage both groups of core muscles.

While everyone could benefit from performing the power push-up exercises in this book, they do provide brilliant advantages to some special populations. For example, if you're someone whose main fitness goal is to gain more power because you're, say, a professional dancer or athlete, then this section will provide that desired power to your entire body. But remember, you don't have to be a professional dancer or world-class athlete to benefit from this power section. Anyone who wants to improve their physical performance and skills, no matter the sport or use of those skills, will experience positive outcomes by performing the power push-ups in this book.

Creating more power is vital because it equates to quickly creating more force to acquire the most muscle fibers possible. For example, walking engages your gluteus maximus muscles only mildly, but performing a jumping jack involves more of your gluteus maxmius muscles. As explained above, we know how crucial it is to have strong gluteal muscles. Traditionally, power movements are explosive exercises that are utilizing heavy force for only one to five repetitions. The power push-up exercises in this book are very different from the "traditional" sense because you are combining all three push-up sections in one. First, you are creating stabilization in your upper body and core muscles during these push-ups. Your shoulders, back, arms, and core stabilization muscles are all engaged to support with stabilization. Second, the act of performing a push-up along with moving the proper core muscles and other muscles in your body is the development of strength. Finally, the power portion of these push-ups is enhanced by the creation of the force you are producing in your upper and lower body.

The rectus abdominis (main core movement muscle) is engaged intensely during the execution of power push-ups due to the forceful movement of the core movement muscles. Therefore, it's possible to work towards obtaining a "six pack" while performing these push-ups. Again, there's no need to waste excessive hours performing an assortment of abdominal exercises, because these power push-ups will engage the rectus abdominis all while saving precious time and energy. Along with the stabilization push-ups and strength push-ups, power push-ups will definitely help you in losing those unwanted pounds for a couple of reasons. First, these power push-ups are unlike the stability and strength push-ups because they promote more cardiovascular ability. Your heart rate will certainly accelerate and stay high during these push-ups because they require more oxygen to perform, hence, more aerobic capacity is needed. Second, as with the other two push-up sections of this book, they will shed unwanted pounds long after you are finished exercising due to safely tearing the muscle fibers, actin and myosin. Performing these power push-up exercises will indisputably assist in building more power, adding more lean mass to your upper body and lower body, engaging your core movement and stabilization muscles, assisting in creating that "six pack," and helping develop more cardiovascular ability.

Progression

This 24 Push-up Journey explains three different fitness levels at which every push-up can be executed. These levels include: beginner, intermediate, and advanced. Each push-up is meticulously designed for the appropriate fitness level based upon sets, repetitions, isometric holds, and rest time. Therefore, please use your best judgement as to which fitness level category presently best defines you. This is a time to be honest with yourself and remember – *you will progress!* The goal is always progression. Especially if you are new to the "fitness world," don't be too aggressive in choosing a fitness level that is more advanced than you might be able to perform. To contrast, if you're someone who exercises constantly and is no stranger to working out, then I absolutely welcome you to engage in a fitness level that is more challenging. In the event that you remain unsure as to which fitness level you should follow, refer to the recommended guidelines below to assist in helping you decide which fitness level is right for you.

Beginner Level

This level is for someone who is either new to exercise or hasn't exercised in some time. This individual might be someone who is sedentary and may have never even performed a push-up before picking up this book. Moreover, the novice could be someone who might have performed push-ups in the past, but may have been performing them incorrectly. A beginner could also be classified as someone who is recovering from an injury and is now eager to get back into a workout routine.

Intermediate Level

This level is for someone who isn't a beginner since this individual does exercise, but just hasn't reached the pinnacle of advanced exercises. This level could include individuals who consistently exercise and have achieved a variety of their own personal fitness goals. On the other hand, the intermediate level could be considered someone who is not incredibly consistent with fitness, however, while working out executes challenging exercises considered more difficult than a beginners' ability.

Advanced Level

This level is for someone who exercises to the highest degree based upon the advanced exercises this individual performs. These exercises include: performing a vast amount of quality repetitions and sets, performing a variety of exercises based upon stability, strength, and power, and exercising consistently for a multitude of months and even years to reach this fitness level. Someone of the advanced level could be considered a professional athlete, "gym rat," or someone who has worked out their entire lives and has made fitness part of their lifestyle. This individual's body is conditioned and their minds are equally as strong when it comes to a challenging workout. The push-ups in this book might be a challenge for someone of this level. Nevertheless, this individual should be trained and experienced enough to be able to attempt this 24 Push-up Journey.

You may be tempted to approach your own push-up journey in the order of your choice. However, I strongly recommend that you complete each push-up section in the order listed for achieving optimal results. Mastering push-ups in terms of stabilization, then strength, to then graduate to power is fundamental in achieving optimal core stabilization and movement muscles while building lean muscle by engaging the correct muscles. Additionally, aim to complete all stabilization, strength, and power push-ups *within your level first,* before upgrading to the next level (in other words, you'll complete all eight push-ups of one level before moving onto the stabilization, strength, and power sections of the next level). Keep in mind, although you may be interested in incorporating some of these push-ups in your current exercise routine, it's best to instill the value of progression with each push-up section and to obtain the most benefits from each individual push-up.

Some of the push-ups in this book may prove to be more of a challenge than others. You may find that you progress steadily in certain sections and more slowly in others. Similarly, you may find that you need more time to fully complete one level before moving onto the next. There's definitely no shame in either scenario; remember that this book is, in fact, a journey, and that just as with any fitness program, your progress is your path. As stated above, patience is crucial even if you happen to hit what's known as a "sticking point." A "sticking point" is referred to as not being able to progress at the same rate of achieving more advanced push-ups than you might have previously once attained. If you happen to get to this point, don't give up or surrender to the more difficult push-ups. You can push past this challenge and progress even if it takes more time than you initially desired. Also, and even more importantly, maintain your motivation as to *why* you are on this push-up journey, and keep the faith even if you happen to become frustrated. Your mind will always outdo your body (unless you have a diagnosed physical limitation) because your body is conditioned to push through even the toughest of physical movements and challenges. Moreover, the body can only do what the mind tells it to perform.

To prevent any regression, be sure you are performing the proper self-care while you partake on this push-up journey. For optimal length-tension relationship in your muscles, remember to stretch the over-active muscles to promote optimal push-up performance. Additionally, proper sleep of seven to eight hours, water intake of two to three liters on exercise days, and a "clean" diet of protein, carbohydrates, and fats are needed as fuel to perform all of these push-ups at your highest capacity.

Remember this is book is a journey and will take time. How long it takes for you is all a part of *your* journey. Aim to perform these push-ups a minimum of once a week, or up to four times a week as your schedule permits. Obviously, with more frequent and correct execution of these push-ups, your abilities should progress to the advanced level. No matter what, remain on your path, and have fun!

Log Your Results

It can be very beneficial to keep records of your push-up journey for multiple reasons. Foremost, regularly tracking your results can help you acknowledge and remember your achievements. It's a wonderful feeling to look back and recall your push-up accomplishments and see how you have progressed. Secondly, think of how much further you will be able to progress on your push-up journey if you're keeping track of your highs and lows. Keeping records of your progress, and even your struggles, can help you define your next goal (whether big or small) by inspiring you to exercise even harder. Lastly, sometimes a number says it all. While performing your push-up routines, writing down the actual number of push-ups you have performed can serve as a gratifying and inspiring reminder. Consider using a notebook, composition book, file on your computer or PDA, or even just a piece of paper; anything that conveniently helps you track and define your results and goals to help keep you going!

Before You Begin

I'd like to take you on a push-up journey. A journey in conquering 24 push-ups for stronger core stabilization and movement muscles, developing more lean muscle in your upper and lower body, and fat loss. This journey will also promote more overall strength, better posture, and provide better function to your muscles. Much like life, this is a journey and not a destination. Bear in mind there is absolutely no timetable or urgency to complete the 24 push-ups immediately. Take your time with these push-ups and take pride with each push-up that you accomplish. There are no inanimate objects needed such as chair, push-up handles, or stability ball when performing these push-ups. The only tools needed on your push-up journey are your own body weight, passionate desire, and consistent patience. Remember that exercising is as much mental as it is physical. Always believe in yourself and your physical abilities. For that reason, before attempting any push-up on your journey, say these words to yourself repeatedly and commit them to your memory, *"I know I can do this push-up."* Positive thoughts are your fuel to succeed even when you feel physically fatigued or doubtful. Moreover, these positive thoughts build mental toughness to not only prosper with each individual push-up in this book, but every activity you personally perform in life. Instead of only passively thinking you are able to perform these push-ups, know in your soul that you can. There is no room for any negative or unconfident thoughts. These judgments only derail you from accomplishing any fitness goal or any other ambition you desire to achieve. Remember always that the mind and the body are needed to work as one functional unit during exercise to yield the best results possible. Believe in the benefits that these push-ups provide. Embrace the challenge for the gratification that exists on the other side. Remember again to have fun and enjoy yourself. *You are doing this for yourself — for you and you alone, to promote better mental and physical health. Now here we go! Embrace the journey!*

PART IV
The 24 Push-up Journey

Stabilization

1. Isometric Push-ups

The first push-up on your journey is an excellent isometric exercise to strengthen your core stabilization muscles and gluteus maximus muscles. The isometric hold will also create lean muscle in your anterior and medial deltoids (front and side shoulders), pectoralis major and minor muscles (chest muscles), and triceps. The back muscles such as your scapulae (shoulder blades) also assist in stabilization to perform the push-up. Moreover, this push-up assists in developing stronger tendons in your rotator cuff.

Starting Position: Begin on the floor, assuming the traditional push-up position with your chest facing downward, legs extended, knees and feet together. Your heels are positioned off the floor and slightly rotated forward. Position your hands slightly more than shoulder-width apart with your elbows only slightly bent.

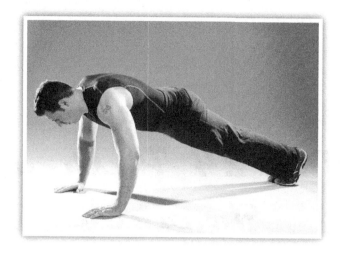

To Perform: Hold this position with your elbows only slightly bent, legs extended, and the knees and feet together. Your heels should still be off the floor and rotated slightly forward. There is no need to lower your upper body downward to the floor at this time since the main goal in this exercise is to achieve more core and upper body stability.

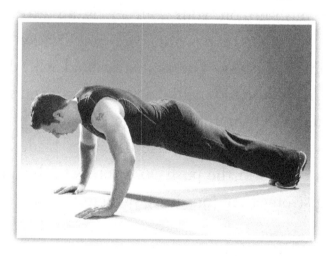

Beginner: Three sets, holding for 10 seconds each
Intermediate: Four sets, holding for 30 seconds each
Advanced: Four sets, holding for 60 seconds each

Rest time between sets should be 30 seconds to one minute for recovery.

Tips: If holding this pose is too difficult, then take the starting position with your legs and feet out wider than shoulder-width apart. This new pose will make it easier for your body to stabilize the hold. However, before moving onto the next push-up, be sure that you can execute this push-up with your knees, legs, and feet together first. Your palms are naturally stable and can provide the proper stability needed to perform this exercise. Therefore, you may use your palms for added stability while performing this push-up, and in doing so alleviate any unwanted strain off of your wrists. Remember to apply "The Focused Five."

2. Isometric Wide-grip Push-ups

This next isometric push-up strengthens your core stabilization muscles, gluteus maximus muscles, anterior and medial deltoids (front and side shoulders), pectoralis major and minor muscles (chest muscles), and triceps. Your scapulae (shoulder blades) are also engaged for stabilization. The isometric hold isolates the medial deltoids due to the wide hand positioning. Additionally, the wider you place your hands, the more you will incorporate your shoulders to create that "broader" look. This exercise will build lean muscle in your upper body due to the time-under-tension from this pose.

Starting Position: Begin by getting into the push-up position with your chest facing downward, legs extended, knees and feet together, and your heels off the floor. Your hands are positioned two steps wider than shoulder-width apart with your elbows only slightly bent.

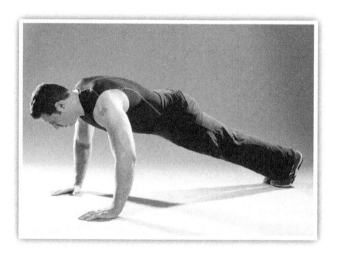

To Perform: Hold this position with your elbows only slightly bent, and the legs extended with knees and feet together. Your heels should be rotated slightly forward. There is no need to lower your upper body to the floor since the main goal in this exercise is to achieve more core and upper body stability.

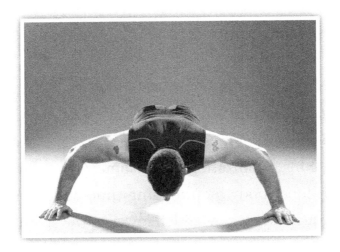

Beginner: Three sets, holding for 10 seconds each
Intermediate: Four sets, holding for 30 seconds each
Advanced: Four sets, holding for 60 seconds each

Rest time between sets should be 30 seconds to one minute for recovery.

Tips: If holding this isometric hold is too difficult, then position your hands only slightly wider than shoulder-width apart. Think of placing your weight on your palms for added assistance in performing this hold. Remember to maintain the neutral spinal position throughout along with continuing to apply "The Focused Five."

3. Isometric Floor Push-ups

This push-up is a nice challenge to strengthen your core stabilization muscles, gluteus maximus muscles, anterior and medial shoulders, pectoralis major and minor muscles, and triceps. Your scapulae muscles are also engaged for stabilization. The isometric hold will build lean muscle in your upper body by providing time-under-tension to your muscles since your body is now much lower to the floor. As such, this push-up also tests your range of motion and provides intense resistance to your muscle fibers. This eccentric (lowest point of range of motion in executing an exercise) hold will also aide in developing stronger tendons to all of your upper body muscles. Moreover, this push-up will strengthen the tendons in your rotator cuffs, while developing even more overall strength to perform more advanced push-ups on your journey. This push-up exercise can also be considered a "shoulder plank."

Starting Position: Begin by getting down on the floor with your chest facing downward with your knees, feet, and legs together with your heels up rotated slightly forward. Your hands are positioned slightly more than shoulder-width apart with your elbows only slightly bent.

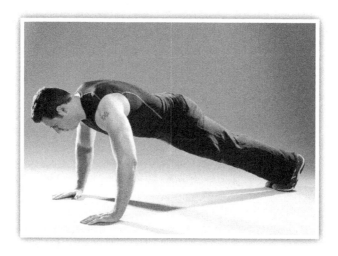

To Perform: Start down on the floor with legs extended, knees and feet together, hands below your shoulders keeping your elbows bent at 90-degrees. Your heels should be off the floor and rotated slightly forward. The overall goal is to lower yourself downward as low as possible with your nose touching the floor, and hold. Your entire body should remain stable throughout.

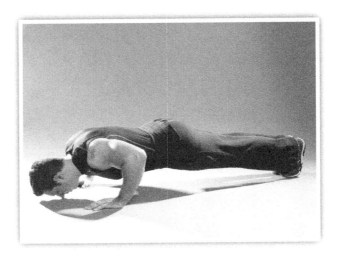

Beginner: Three sets, holding for 10 seconds each
Intermediate: Four sets, holding for 30 seconds each
Advanced: Four sets, holding for 60 seconds each

Rest time between sets should be two to three minutes for recovery.

Tips: If holding this position is too difficult, then only lower your body downward as low as you are able without breaking correct form. Lowering your body even slightly will develop stability and strength to perform more advanced push-ups. Your elbows should be bent at 90-degrees while holding this isometric pose, however, do not have your elbows flair outward beyond 90-degrees since this could cause unnecessary strain to your shoulders and elbows. Maintain stability in your palms to help assist the shoulders and triceps while lowering your body downward to the floor. Remember to utilize "The Focused Five."

4. Isometric Staggered Push-ups

This is an advanced isometric exercise since it incorporates more shoulder and triceps stability than the Traditional Push-up, and therefore, incorporates more strength in your core and rotator cuffs. This exercise builds lean muscle in the anterior and medial deltoid muscles, pectoralis major and pectoralis minor muscles, triceps, and gluteus maximus muscles. Moreover, this "staggered" position will help aide in creating more overall stability in your scapulae muscles. Having more stability in your scapulae muscles aides in shoulder strength to perform pressing movements with functional efficiency.

Starting Position: Begin with your arms in a traditional push-up position, but then stagger your hands by moving one upwards (away from your shoulders) about six inches, and the other downwards (towards your waist) about six inches, keeping them slightly wider than shoulder-width apart. Your legs are extended, and your knees and and feet should stay together with your heels up and your body weight forward on your hands, all of which create more resistance to the upper body.

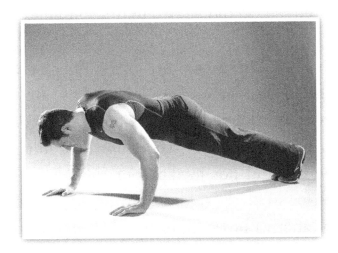

To Perform: Hold this staggered position with your hands while lowering your body to the floor keeping your knees, feet, and legs together. Your upper body and lower body should lower downward together as one unit. Your heels should be off the floor and rotated slightly forward.

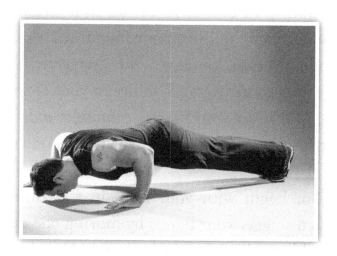

Beginner: Four sets total, two sets each side, holding for 15 seconds each
Intermediate: Six sets total, three sets each side, holding for 30 seconds each
Advanced: Six sets total, three sets each side, holding for 60 seconds each

Rest time between sets should be two to three minutes for recovery.

Tips: If lowering yourself downward to the floor proves to be too challenging, then lower yourself as low as you are able without breaking correct form. Remember: it's vital to maintain the neutral spinal position while not hiking your hips or leaning to one side throughout. Be mindful not to dip your shoulder or elevate your upper trapezius for strength. Additionally, if placing your hands six inches from one another proves to be too challenging, you may bring them closer for added stability.

5. Isometric One-Leg Push-ups

The first four isometric push-up exercises on your journey engaged more of the core stabilization muscles by keeping the legs, knees, and feet together in a variety of different hand positions. After completing these previous exercises, this isometric push-up now involves the lower body, and therefore challenges the core in a new difficult way by engaging the core movement muscles, such as the erector spinae. This isometric push-up builds lean muscle in the primary movers of this exercise, which are: the anterior and medial deltoid muscles, pectoralis major and pectoralis minor muscles, triceps, gluteus maximus muscle, quadriceps, hamstrings, and calves.

Starting Position: Position your hands in the traditional push-up position. Your chest is facing the floor and your elbows are only slightly bent. Next, bring one leg only a few inches off the floor while your other foot remains stationary with the heel up. The leg that is in the air is locked at the knee for more hamstring and gluteus maximus muscle recruitment.

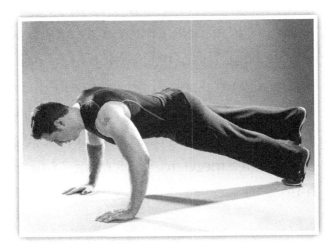

To Perform: Lower your body downward in a controlled manner while keeping the leg that is in the air stationary throughout with little-to-no movement. The leg supporting your body should also be locked (extended) at the knee throughout. For optimal range of motion, your nose should gently touch the floor while holding.

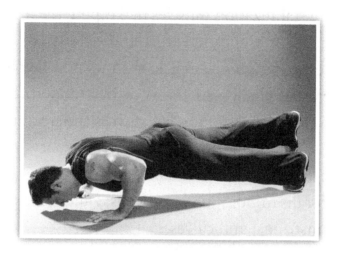

Beginner: Six sets total, three sets each side, holding for 10 seconds
Intermediate: Six sets total, three sets each side, holding for 30 seconds
Advanced: Six sets total, three sets each side, holding for one minute

Rest time between sets should be two to three minutes for recovery.

Tips: Be mindful not to raise the leg that is up more than a few inches from the floor. Doing so is incorrect form and could result in causing unnecessary strain to your lower back. Moreover, doing so hinders your ability to obtain a neutral spinal position and therefore does not engage proper core movement and stabilization muscles. Be mindful to not lean or hike your hips during this push-up, too, especially while holding one leg up. Don't forget to implement "The Focused Five" during this push-up!

6. Isometric Side Leg Extension Push-ups

This isometric push-up builds lean muscle in the primary movers of this exercise, which are the anterior and medial deltoid muscles, pectoralis major and pectoralis minor muscles, triceps, gluteus maximus muscle, gluteus minimus, gluteus medius, quadriceps, hamstrings, and calves. This exercise also provides an incredible static stretch to your hip flexor and psoas major muscles.

Starting Position: Place your hands in the traditional push-up position. Your chest is facing the floor and your elbows are only slightly bent. Your legs are locked, your knees and feet are together with your heels slightly pushed forward.

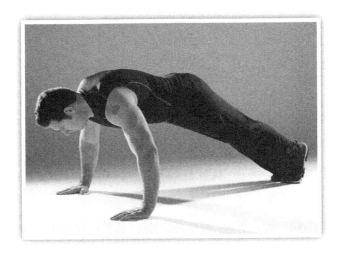

To Perform: Lower your body downward in a controlled manner as you raise one leg upward (away from the floor), and then out to the side (away from the body) at hip-level.

For optimal range of motion in your upper body, your nose should delicately touch the floor. Your other foot remains stationary with the heel up. The leg that is in the air is locked (extended) at the knee for more hamstring and gluteus maximus, gluteus minimus, and gluteus medius muscle recruitment. Your raised leg should be positioned six inches out to the side from the starting position for optimal range of motion during this isometric hold. The supporting leg should also be locked at the knee throughout. When finished, bring your leg back carefully into the starting position.

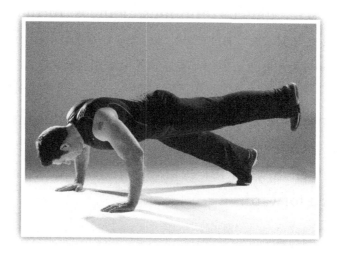

Beginner: Six sets total, three sets, holding for 10 seconds each
Intermediate: Six sets total, three sets, holding for 30 seconds each
Advanced: Six sets total, three sets, holding for one minute each

Rest time between sets should be two to three minutes for recovery.

Tips: Be mindful not to raise the leg that is in the air out from the spine more than your spine can handle. A good guide to keep the correct form is to be sure that you are not leaning excessively or hiking your hips. This incorrect form might create unnecessary strain to your lower back that could result in injury. Again, performing any of these push-ups with incorrect form can result in losing the neutral spinal position and therefore does not the engage the correct core movement and core stabilization muscles.

7. Isometric Alternating Knee-to-Chest Leg Flexion Push-ups

This next push-up exercise will challenge you differently from the others since your upper body will provide stabilization while your lower body is in movement. This is more difficult than the other previous isometric push-up exercises because of the duration of time it takes to complete a full set. This lower body movement could be considered a "slow moving mountain climber" since you are performing the same range of motion as a mountain climber, but with slower frequency. You will produce lean muscle in your gluteus maximus muscle, hamstrings, quadriceps, and calves. Other primary movers in the upper body during this exercise are: anterior and medial deltoid muscles, pectoralis major and pectoralis minor muscles, and triceps.

Starting Position: Begin with your chest facing the floor with your hands slightly more than shoulder-width apart. The legs are extended with knees and feet together to promote optimal core stability with your heels slightly rotated forward.

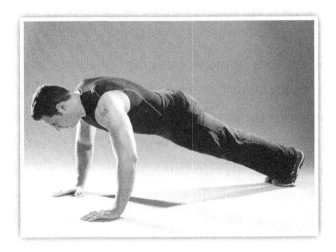

To Perform: Lower yourself into a push-up with your nose gently touching the floor. While holding this position, keep your elbows bent at 90-degrees and bend one knee, bringing it up towards your chest slowly while your other foot remains stationary on the floor with your heel up. Then repeat the same action with your other leg. Performing one push-up and two knee-to-chest leg flexion movements with each leg equals one full repetition.

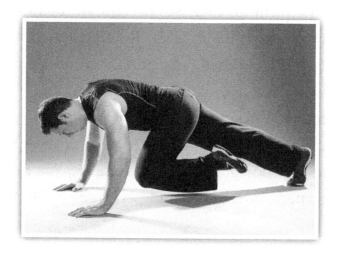

Beginner: Three sets total, 10 repetitions each
Intermediate: Four sets total, 16 repetitions each
Advanced: Four sets total, 20 repetitions each

Rest time between sets should be two to three minutes for full recovery.

Tips: If you're having trouble staying all the way down while performing the lower body movements, rise up slightly to make this exercise less challenging. Be especially diligent while performing the knee to chest flexion portion of this push-up. The stabilization portion of this exercise comes from the time-under-tension that this exercise provides, and therefore, they should be done *slowly*. Range of motion is critical too when executing the knee to chest flexion exercise. Your knee should aim to touch the bottom of your chest for each repetition. As always, maintain a neutral spinal position during this push-up and do not be tempted to round your back, especially while flexing your knee towards your chest. Don't forget "The Focused Five!"

8. Isometric T-Rotation Push-ups

Your stabilization journey is almost complete, as you have now approached the final isometric push-up exercise! All of the other previous isometric stabilization push-up exercises have prepared you for this last stabilization exercise before continuing your journey onto the strength section. This final push-up requires an abundance of shoulder, triceps, rotator cuff, hip flexor, erector spinae, and most importantly, core stabilization muscles along with some core movement muscles. Moreover, this exercise requires optimal rotation in activating your internal and external obliques. This isometric push-up builds lean muscle in your gluteus maximus muscles, hamstrings, quadriceps, and calves. Other primary movers in this exercise are: anterior and medial deltoid muscles, pectoralis major and pectoralis minor muscles, and triceps.

Starting Position: Begin with your chest facing the floor with your hands slightly more than shoulder-width apart. Your legs are locked with knees and feet together to promote optimal core stability.

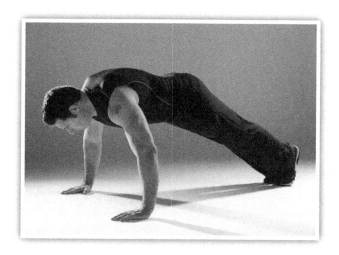

To Perform: Lower yourself down about halfway from the floor and then begin to rise up towards the starting position. As you raise your body upward, begin to push off with one arm and rotate your entire body to one side. The arm on the side in which you are rotating will become extended at your elbow forming a "T" shape while your other arm remains extended supporting your body weight. Both of your feet will be fully rotated and on top of one another for optimal core stabilization and core movement muscle recruitment.

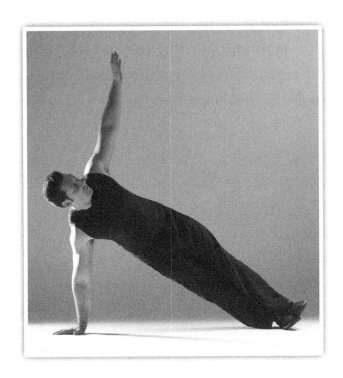

Beginner: Three sets total, eight repetitions total (four repetitions each side without alternating), and holding the T-position for five seconds
Intermediate: Three sets total, 12 repetitions total (six repetitions each side without alternating), and holding the T-position for five seconds
Advanced: Three sets total, 12 repetitions total (six repetitions each side without alternating), and holding the T-position for 10 seconds

Rest time between sets should be two to three minutes for full recovery.

Tips: Remember there is no need to lower all the way down since the main objective of this push-up is to create stability and tendon strength. If this exercise is too difficult to perform with one leg on top of the other than you may place one foot on the floor in front of your other foot. This will create added stability while keeping the integrity of the important "T" position in your arms. Be sure to extend your arm fully while performing the T-position for optimal resistance for your core stabilization muscles and upper body. As always, maintain a neutral spinal position during this push-up by not dropping the hip on the same side as the supporting arm, but keeping it aligned with your shoulder. Remember "The Focused Five" here, since you'll need all of your muscles to help accordingly.

STRENGTH

1. Traditional Push-ups

After successfully conquering all of the previous isometric stabilization push-ups, it's time to attempt the ever-popular Traditional Push-up. Before even attempting this push-up, *do not be consumed with how far you are able to lower your body down.* That range of motion and overall strength will certainly develop as you progress on your journey. For now, focus on your breath (for added strength), engage your core stabilization muscles and gluteus maximus muscles, and embrace the challenge your own body weight provides. Remember that you are now pushing your own body weight, as this is the first push-up in the foundation to build strength. This exercise builds lean muscle in these primary movers: anterior and medial deltoid muscles, pectoralis major and pectoralis minor muscles, triceps, and gluteus maximus. Also, your latissimus dorsi muscles and scapulae muscles are engaged for added stability.

Starting Position: Position yourself with your chest facing the floor with your hands a little more than shoulder-width apart. Your legs are locked, with knees and feet together to promote optimal core stability. Your heels should be positioned slightly forward for added resistance to engage more of your upper body.

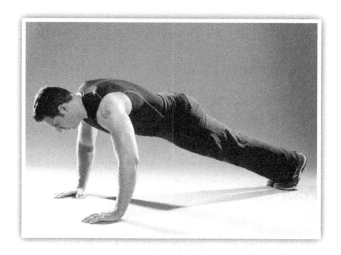

To Perform: Lower yourself downward while bending your elbows at 90 degrees in a controlled fashion and pause briefly before raising yourself up back to the starting position. Don't forget your breath for added strength! Do your best to eventually have your nose gently touch the floor for optimal range of motion.

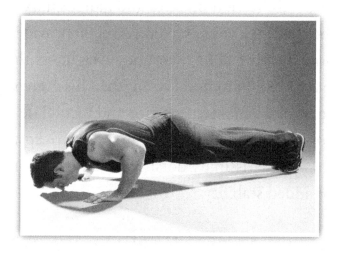

Beginners: Three sets of 10 repetitions each
Intermediate: Four sets of 20 repetitions each
Advanced: Four sets of 30 repetitions each

Rest time between sets should be one to three minutes for recovery.

Tips: If this exercise proves to be too difficult, remember to please be patient with your range of motion and stay consistent. With consistency and proper form, you will eventually obtain the proper strength to have your nose gently touch the floor. Again, your elbows should not flair outward more than 90 degrees since this could cause unnecessary strain to your elbows and shoulders. Be mindful that positioning your feet in a shoulder-width stance would make this exercises incredibly easier, but isn't as beneficial in developing the core movement and stabilization muscles. Also, at this point of your journey, not keeping your feet together would only decrease your progression to perform other push-ups effectively. Remember to shift your weight from your wrists to your palms for added stability. Continue to apply "The Focused Five."

2. Staggered Push-Ups

This is an advanced exercise since it incorporates more core, shoulder, and triceps stability than the Traditional Push-up, and therefore incorporates more strength in your rotator cuffs. This push-up builds lean muscle in the primary movers of this exercise which are the: anterior and medial deltoid muscles, pectoralis major and pectoralis minor muscles, triceps, and gluteus maximus muscle. Moreover, the "staggered" position of your hands will help in creating more overall strength when performing other push-ups that otherwise start with your hands shoulder-width apart.

Starting Position: Begin with your arms in a traditional push-up position, but then stagger your hands by moving one upwards about six inches (away from the shoulder), and the other downwards (towards your waist) about six inches, keeping them shoulder-width apart. Your legs are locked, knees and feet are together with your heels up and your body weight forward on your hands, all of which create a more challenging core workout.

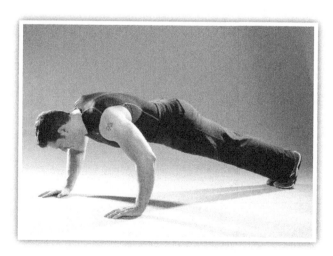

To Perform: Once you rise up from one push-up, continue to execute the next repetition while keeping your core in the neutral spinal position. The optimal goal is to have your gently nose touch the floor with every repetition. The elbow that is forward should be bent at 90-degrees while your rear elbow is bent at 40-degrees.

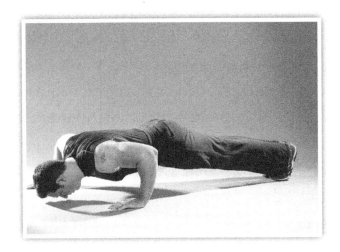

Beginners: Four sets total, two sets each side of 10 repetitions
Intermediate: Six sets total, three sets each side of 16 repetitions
Advanced: Six sets total, three sets each side of 24 repetitions

Rest time between sets should be two to three minutes for recovery.

Tips: Particularly while performing this push-up, it's vital to maintain the neutral spinal position for engaging optimal core movement muscles. If you happen to lean with your hips or hike your hips up, this core positioning would not engage the correct core muscles. Be mindful to not dip your shoulder or elevate your upper trapezius for strength. If the starting position proves to be too challenging, you may bring your hands in (closer towards the shoulders) for added stability. However, when that position proves comfortable or easy, challenge yourself by bringing them out to a true six inches apart before moving forward in your push-up journey.

3. One-Leg Staggered Push-Ups

The first three push-up exercises engaged more of the core stabilization muscles by keeping the legs, knees, and feet together. After conquering them, this next push-up gets the lower body involved, and thus, challenges the core in a new, demanding way by engaging more of the core movement muscles such as the erector spinae. This push-up builds lean muscle in the primary movers of this exercise, which are the anterior and medial deltoid muscles, pectoralis major and pectoralis minor muscles, triceps, gluteus maximus muscle, quadriceps, hamstrings, and calves. Your latissimus dorsi and scapulae muscles are also engaged.

Starting Position: Begin with your arms in a traditional push-up position, but then stagger your hands by moving one upwards about six inches, and the other downwards about six inches, keeping them shoulder-width apart. Your chest is facing the floor and your elbows are only slightly bent. Next, if your right hand is forward in the staggered position, then raise your right leg only a few inches off the floor while your other foot remains stationary with the heel up. The leg that is in the air is locked at the knee for more hamstring and gluteus maximus muscle recruitment.

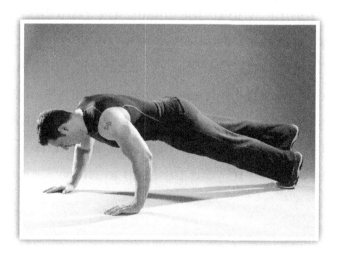

To Perform: Lower your body downward in a controlled manner while keeping the leg that is in the air stationary throughout with little to no movement. The leg supporting your body should also be locked (extended) at the knee throughout. For optimal range of motion, your nose should gently touch the floor.

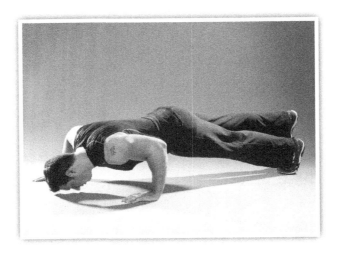

Beginner: Six sets total, two sets each side of 12 repetitions
Intermediate: Six sets total, three sets each side of 16 repetitions
Advanced: Six sets total, three sets each side of 24 repetitions

Rest time between sets should be two to three minutes for recovery.

Tips: Remember that if your right leg is in the air then your right hand is positioned forward in the staggered position. This positioning in your upper body and lower body recruits more of the core movement muscles such as your latissimus dorsi. To contrast, if your left hand was forward in the staggered position with your right leg in air, this positioning would not create optimal core muscle recruitment. Be mindful not to raise the leg that is up more than a few inches from the floor. This is incorrect form and could cause unnecessary strain to your lower back. Additionally, doing so impedes your ability to obtain a neutral spinal position and therefore does not recruit proper core movement and stabilization muscles. Be mindful to not lean or hike up your hips during this push-up, too, especially while holding one leg up.

4. Alternating Side Extension Push-ups

It's time to progress your leg movements with a more challenging movement pattern for your core. This new leg movement is the side extension. The side leg extension engages the core movement muscles and activates your hip adductors and hip abductor muscles. This push-up will build lean muscle in your anterior and medial deltoid muscles, pectoralis major and pectoralis minor muscles, triceps, gluteus maximus muscle, gluteus medius muscles, quadriceps, hamstrings, and calves.

Starting Position: Begin with your arms in a traditional push-up position with your elbows slightly bent, chest facing the floor. Your legs are locked, with knees and feet together, and weight on the balls of your feet.

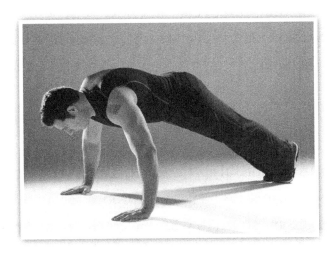

To Perform: Lower your body downward in a controlled manner while you bring one leg out to the side with your knee extended (locked) at hip-level. For optimal range of motion, your nose should gently touch the floor during each push-up. Your raised leg should be moved six inches out to the side. The leg supporting your body should also be locked at the knee throughout. Next, rise up back into the starting position while simultaneously bringing your leg back to center, with your upper body and lower body moving as one unit. One push-up with one side leg extension equals one repetition. Continue to execute a push-up while alternating your legs outward to the side to complete a set.

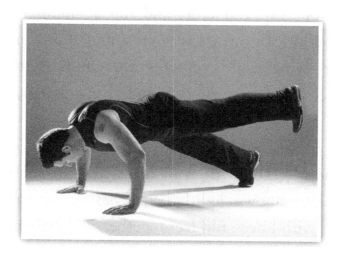

Beginner: Six sets total, three sets each side, 10 repetitions
Intermediate: Six sets total, three sets each side, 16 repetitions
Advanced: Six sets total, three sets each side, 24 repetitions

Rest time between sets should be two to three minutes for recovery.

Tips: Be mindful to not raise the leg that is in the air higher than hip-level throughout because this is improper form and could result in causing unnecessary strain to your lower back. Furthermore, doing so hinders your ability to keep the neutral spinal position, and thus does not engage the correct core movement and stabilization muscles. Also, do not drop your leg that is in the air lower than hip-level because it will disengage your core movement muscles. Remember to not lean or hike your hips during this push-up, either, especially while holding your leg up. Remember to apply "The Focused Five" to maximize all of their benefits!

5. X Push-ups

This push-up provides a different challenge in your journey than all of the other previous strength push-up exercises because you will be executing movement with your arms. Performing push-ups with hand movements while your legs are stable is much more challenging than performing push-up exercises while your arms are stable with leg movements. This is due to the core stabilization and movement muscles correctly engaging to perform the exercise for optimal efficiency. The X Push-up is a nice challenge to introduce arm movements due to your lower body moving with your upper body. The "X" movement of this push-up will add extra stability for the core and make this portion of the push-up easier to perform while engaging your hip abductors. However, the constant movement in your upper and lower body will be a great test for your core movement muscles. This push-up builds lean muscle in the primary movers such as the anterior and medial deltoid muscles, pectoralis major and pectoralis minor muscles, triceps, and all three of your gluteal muscles. Your latissimus dorsi muscles and scapulae provide extra stability during this exercise.

Starting position: Start with your hands and feet positioned two steps wider than your traditional push-up position. This creates the "X" that your upper and lower body will be forming throughout this push-up exercise.

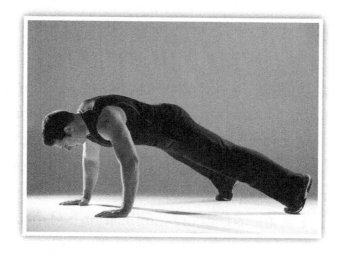

To Perform: Lower yourself downward into a push-up with your elbows bent at 90-degrees with your nose gently touching the floor. Then, rise up back into the starting position and bring your knees, legs, and feet together. Next, move your hands inward to shoulder-width apart as you then execute another push-up with your elbows bent at 40-degrees, with your nose gently touching the floor. Continue to move your upper and lower body back into the "X" position and perform a push-up while moving your upper and lower body back into the close position. Develop a consistent tempo or speed in completing these two push-up movements. The optimal goal is to have your nose touch the floor for both of these push-ups for optimal range of motion.

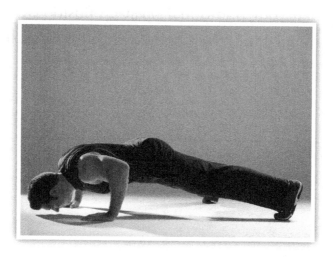

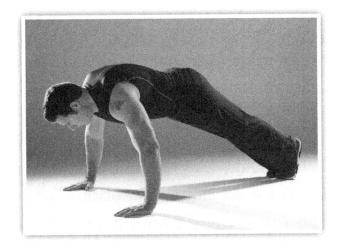

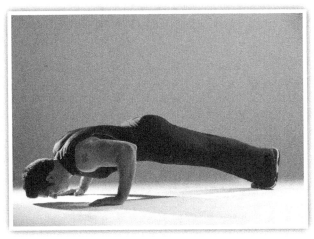

Beginner: Three sets total, one set equals performing both push-ups for 10 repetitions

Intermediate: Four sets total, one set equals performing both push-ups for 16 repetitions

Advanced: Four sets total, one set equals performing both push-ups for 24 repetitions

Rest time between sets should be two to three minutes for recovery.

Tips: Remember to stay controlled during this exercise, especially when it comes to moving your arms, and place your hands down gently on the floor throughout. It's vital to keep the neutral spinal position throughout since both your upper and lower body are in motion to avoid any lower back strain in the erector spinae. The X portion of this push-up should feel easier than the second portion of this exercise due to less core stability needed to perform the push-up. Although, if this exercise proves to be too difficult, position your hands greater than shoulder-width apart with your knees, legs, and feet together during the second portion of this push-up for added stability. Remember to use your palms, not your wrists, for added stability when executing these push-ups. Continue to be mindful of engaging the "Focused Five" throughout this exercise.

6. Slap Push-ups

After completely the previous push-up with hand movements, you are now ready for an even more advanced challenge in your push-up journey by only moving your arms while keeping your lower body stable throughout. This push-up, if executed correctly, is extremely difficult since it's a functional challenge as much as a strength training exercise. Notably, when arm movements are involved in push-ups the core stabilization and movement muscles must correctly perform the exercise for optimal efficiency. It's especially easy to perform with inefficient form. This exercise will provide a tremendous amount of shoulder, triceps, and rotator cuff stability. It also challenges your hip flexors and psoas muscles since there can be absolutely no leaning to either side. This push-up also creates lean muscle in the primary movers such as the anterior and medial deltoid muscles, pectoralis major and pectoralis minor muscles, triceps, and gluteus maximus muscle with your latissimus dorsi and scapulae muscles engaged.

Starting position: As with the above techniques, keep your knees, legs, and feet together to engage your core and maintain a neutral spinal position in your back. Next, place your hands slightly more than shoulder-width apart.

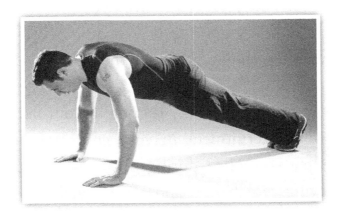

To Perform: Lower into a traditional push-up and as you lift your body up from the floor to return to the starting push-up position, quickly "slap" one hand on your opposite shoulder and return your hand back to the floor to stabilize your body. Next, execute another push-up descending your body towards the floor and repeat the slap with the opposite hand at the top of the push-up. Develop a consistent and controlled tempo in executing these alternating sides movements. The optimal goal is to have your nose gently touch the floor with each push-up for optimal range of motion. Performing one push-up and one slap movement is considered one repetition.

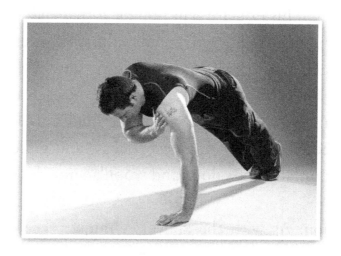

Beginner: Three sets total, 10 repetitions each
Intermediate: Four sets total, 16 repetitions each
Advanced: Four sets total, 20 repetitions each

Rest time between sets should be two to three minutes for recovery.

Tips: The goal is to not allow any leaning in your body or any hip hiking for optimal recruitment in your core movement muscles. Remember to stay controlled during this exercise especially when it comes to moving your hands, and place your hands down gently on the floor throughout. If this exercise proves to be too difficult, position your hands greater than shoulder-width apart. This position will create more stabilization and engage more secondary muscles for support. Again, use your palms for added stabilization and do not hesitate when performing the slap touches. Remember to utilize "The Focused Five" during this exercise.

7. Push-Ups with Reach

Much like the Slap Push-up and the Staggered Moving Push-up, this is an even more advanced exercise that challenges the core movement muscles for optimal efficiency because one arm will be stabilizing your body weight for a longer period of time than the preceding push-ups. This exercise creates a tremendous amount of stability in the upper body, and therefore strength in your rotator cuffs, shoulders, and triceps. This push-up, much like the previous two mentioned above, challenges your hip flexors and psoas muscles since there can be absolutely no leaning. This push-up also creates lean muscle in the primary movers such as the: anterior and medial deltoid muscles, pectoralis major and pectoralis minor muscles, triceps, and gluteus maximus muscle. Your latissimus dorsi, rhomboids, and scapulae muscles are also engaged during this push-up.

Starting Position: To begin, start in the traditional push-up position with your knees, feet, and legs together. Your hands should be positioned slightly more than shoulder-width apart.

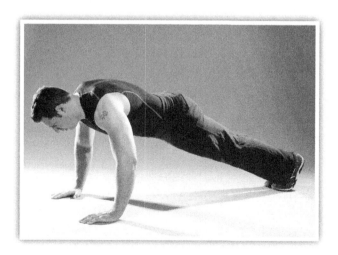

To Perform: Lower downward into a push-up with your nose touching the floor. Then, as you rise up to the starting position slowly, without leaning or hiking your hips, extend to one arm fully upward off the floor while locking your elbow at shoulder-level. Place your hand down to the floor in a controlled fashion and then repeat with your other arm on the other side. Performing one push-up and extending both arms outward is one repetition.

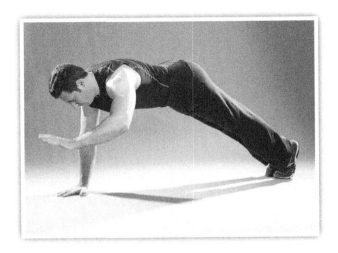

Beginner: Three sets total, eight repetitions
Intermediate: Four sets total, 12 repetitions
Advanced: Four sets total, 16 repetitions

Rest time between sets should be two to three minutes for recovery.

Tips: Again, for optimal core movement muscle and core stabilization muscle recruitment there must be little-to-no movement in your hips. This is incredibly difficult especially on the side on which you are over-active (tighter) while stabilizing you. (To specify, if you are right dominant, when the right hand is on the floor and your left arm is extended at shoulder-level, this has traditionally proven to be more challenging.) Thus, continue to bend your elbows and take each repetition slowly throughout to help maintain stability in your hips. Remember to "reset" if needed in the starting position by fully engaging your correct core muscles and your gluteus maximus muscles for added strength before you perform this push-up. Continue to apply "The Focused Five!"

8. Plank-ups with Push-ups

At this point of your push-up journey, it's definitely time to celebrate your push-up accomplishments! You have obviously successfully completed all of the Stabilization Push-up exercises and are currently on the verge to finishing the last of the Strength Push-up exercises. In your current journey, you have mastered numerous hand and leg positioning movements, which have all been a different test for your core muscles. The Plank-ups with Push-ups exercise should be more of a challenge than all of the previous exercises. One factor is now you will be exercising in two different planes of motion for the first time on your journey. Push-ups are performed in the transverse plane of motion or also known as the horizontal plane. In contrast, planks are performed in the sagittal plane. Performing exercises in two different planes of motion especially when supersetting (performing back-to-back exercises with no rest) can be very difficult on your muscles, as well as to the central nervous system since these are unknown movements. Hence, this push-up is the ultimate exercise for creating paramount engagement of the core stabilization and movement muscles. This push-up creates lean muscle in the primary movers such as the anterior and medial deltoid muscles, pectoralis major and pectoralis minor muscles, triceps, and gluteus maximus muscle. Your forearms, latissimus dorsi, rhomboids, and scapulae muscles are also engaged during this exercise.

Starting Position: As with most of the beginning push-up positions above, start in the traditional push-up position with your knees, feet, and legs together. Your hands should be positioned slightly more than shoulder-width apart.

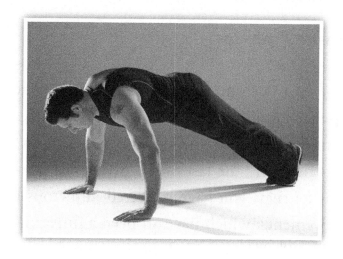

To Perform: Lower your body downward into a push-up keeping your knees, feet, and legs together with your nose gently touching the floor. Then after performing the push-up, return to the starting position keeping your arms and legs in the same position. Next, lower yourself into the plank position with both of your forearms on the floor. Your forearms should be aligned with your anterior shoulders. Be mindful of what arm you brought downward first into the plank position since that will be the same arm that will lead into bringing you back into the starting position. For example, if you brought your left arm downward first into the plank position followed by your right arm, then the left hand will propel you upward first with your right hand following. It's critical that you maintain the order of movement on what arm is leading during this push-up. Finish this exercise by rising upward back into the starting position with your hands positioned slightly wider than shoulder-width. Performing one push-up and one plank-up is considered one repetition.

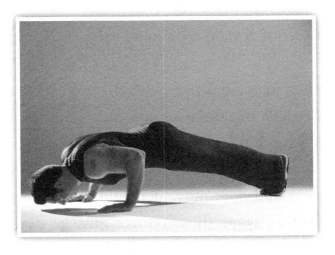

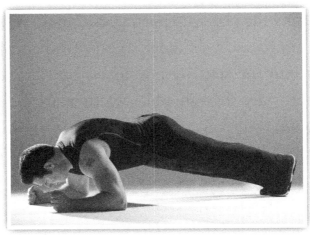

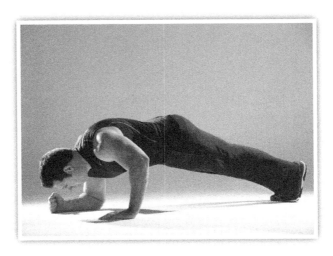

Beginner: Three sets, 10 repetitions total, five repetitions each side
Intermediate: Three sets, 16 repetitions, eight repetitions each side
Advanced: Three sets, 20 repetitions, 10 repetitions each side

Rest time between sets should be two to three minutes for recovery.

Tips: Remember to maintain a neutral spinal position during this exercise. Be cautious not to create too much hip hiking, leaning, or movement in your hips after performing the plank-up portion of this exercise because otherwise you are not engaging the optimal core stabilization and core movement muscles. Therefore, take this exercise *slowly* and engage those correct muscles needed to perform this exercise more efficiently. Although, do your best not too hesitate very much during the plank-up portion during this exercise since this could create unnecessary shoulder strain or other injuries. If rising upward back into the starting position is too difficult, then bring your hands out wider than shoulder-width apart for added stability. You may also use your palms for added stability during the push-up of this exercise. Continue to remember the "Focused Five" since these helpful tools are the foundation to correct your form for any push-up.

POWER

1. Alternating Leg Push-Ups

This push-up starts your journey into the final section of this book. This exercise is a power movement that will involve more of your lower body since you will begin to implement jumping movements while building stronger core movement muscles and stabilization muscles in the process. This push-up builds lean muscle in the primary movers of this exercise which are the anterior and medial deltoid muscles, pectoralis major and pectoralis minor muscles, triceps, gluteus maximus muscle, quadriceps, hamstrings, and calves. Your latissimus dorsi and scapulae are still helping stabilize during this exercise. Since this is a power movement, practically every muscle below your pelvis will be stretched during this exercise due to the height of your lower body.

Starting Position: Begin by getting into the push-up position with your hands positioned slightly wider than shoulder-width apart. You will have one leg up extended (locked) at the knee about two inches from the floor with your other foot on the floor.

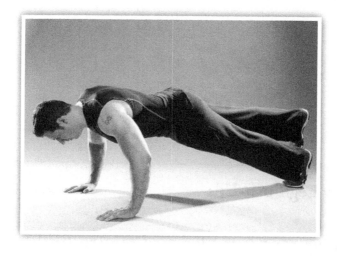

To Perform: With one leg up about two inches above the floor, lower your body downward, executing a push-up. The leg that is in the air is locked (extended) at the knee to recruit more muscle fibers in your gluteal muscles and hamstring. Before you begin the next repetition, alternate legs by raising the other leg two inches above the floor, with a hop to the motion as you switch legs. This "hop" will provide the power needed in this exercise. Do not bring the raised leg higher than two inches above the floor because bringing your legs too high could cause unwanted strain and possible injury to your lower back muscles. The optimal goal is to have your nose gently touch the floor with each push-up for optimal range of motion while keeping constant form in your lower body. To clarify, one repetition equals one push-up with one leg up.

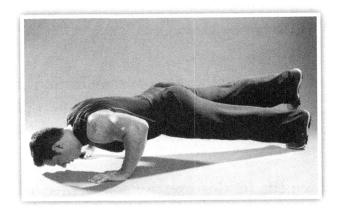

Beginner: Three sets, 10 repetitions (five with each leg)
Intermediate: Four sets, 12 repetitions (six with each leg)
Advanced: Four sets, 20 repetitions (10 with each leg)

Rest time between sets should be two to four minutes for recovery.

Tips: As stated above, be vigilant to not raise the raised leg more than a few inches from the floor. Raising it too high can jeopardize the crucial neutral spinal position needed in this exercise for optimal engagement of the core movement and core stabilization muscles. Do your best to maintain the power needed for proper execution in this movement by starting the "hopping" motion as you rise up from the push-up. Remember as always not to lean or hike your hips upwards while performing this powerful movement. Lastly, do not drop your shoulder or elevate your upper trapezius. Engage your gluteus maximus muscles, "draw in" your abdominals for strength, perform correct breathing, and utilize the rest of "The Focused Five" as you perform this push-up.

2. In-to-Out Push-ups

This is an advanced exercise for the core stabilization and movement muscles because it incorporates arms movements that move from side-to-side with extreme hand placement.

The power movement in this exercise is executed in your hands; therefore, do not "drag" your hands along the floor during this exercise. You will bring your hands off the floor while creating extreme speed for the proper power needed in this exercise. Note that creating excessive height while performing these hand movements is not required during this push-up. This exercise creates a large amount of shoulder and triceps stability from the first-to-final repetition due to its hand positioning. This push-up builds lean muscle in the primary movers such as the anterior and medial deltoid muscles, pectoralis major and pectoralis minor muscles, triceps, and gluteus maximus muscle. At this point of the push-up journey, your core stabilization and movement muscles are strong, and therefore, they will assist with the shoulder and triceps strength needed for optimal performance.

Starting Position: Position yourself with your chest facing the floor with your hands positioned close to one another. Your knees, legs, and feet are together with your toes positioned slightly forward.

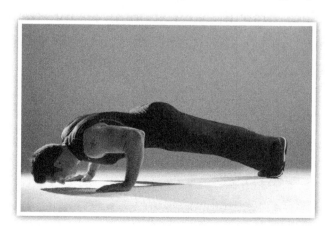

To Perform: Start by executing a push-up with your hands close to one another and then rise up back into the starting position. Next, slightly move your hands out horizontally while increasing speed, bringing your hands slightly off the floor. Continue to perform three more push-ups while placing your hands a few more inches apart in between each repetition. After performing four repetitions (push-ups), your hands should be positioned more than shoulder-width apart. To finish a completed round, keep on executing a push-up while bringing your hands in a few inches with every repetition until you are back at starting position. If accomplished correctly, you should execute four push-ups out and then four push-ups in for one full round. As with all push-ups, the paramount goal is to have your nose safely touch the floor for optimal range of motion.

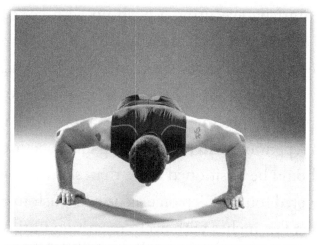

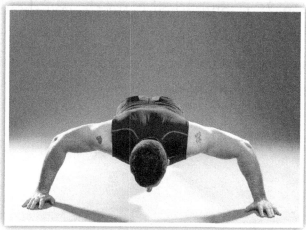

Beginners: Three sets total, one set is considered two rounds of performing four push-ups out and then four push-ups in.

Intermediate: Three sets total, one set is considered three rounds of performing four push-ups out and then four push-ups in.

Advanced: Three sets total, one set is considered four rounds of performing four push-ups out and then four push-ups in.

Rest time between sets should be two to four minutes for recovery.

Tips: Be mindful not to place your hands more than a few inches apart while performing every push-up. The core stabilization and core movement muscles activate more efficiently with smaller shifts in hand placements. As with other strength exercises you have previously performed, do not hesitate during this exercise during the hand placements since this could cause unnecessary strain to your rotator cuffs and shoulders. Again, there is no need to create extreme height with your hands while moving them inward and outward. The power in this exercise is implemented with the speed that you are creating between each push-up. That said, maintain a neutral spinal position throughout, especially when bringing your hands outward past your shoulders. All of your core muscles and gluteus maximus muscles should be engaged throughout for added ability to perform this push-up. Apply "The Focused Five!"

3. Staggered Moving Hand Push-ups

This is an advanced exercise for the core stabilization and core movement muscles since it incorporates staggered arm movements in your upper body. The power in this exercise is once again executed in your hand positioning by generating constant speed. Again, push-ups become significantly more challenging when your arms and hands are in motion. As with any staggered position push-up, this is a beneficial exercise for shoulder, triceps, and rotator cuff stability. This push-up builds lean muscle in the primary movers of this exercise which are the: anterior and medial deltoid muscles, pectoralis major and pectoralis minor muscles, triceps, and gluteus maximus muscle. Your latissimus dorsi and other back muscles are assisting with stabilization during this exercise. Much like the Slap Push-up, this particular exercise challenges the hip flexors and psoas muscles not to lean, creating optimal core stabilization and core movement muscles.

Starting Position: Begin with your arms in a traditional push-up position, but then stagger your hands by moving one upwards about six inches, and the other downwards about six inches, keeping them slightly more than shoulder-width apart. Your knees, legs, and feet should all be together while your heels are up rotated slightly forward.

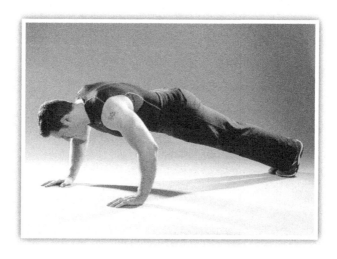

To Perform: From one push-up to the next, alternate the hands in the staggered position at the height of the push-up, gently moving your hands on the floor in between each repetition. Do not perform a dragging motion with your hands on the floor, nor do you need to create a hop with your hands during this exercise. This push-up will be a challenge by creating the wide range of motion in your hand positioning by keeping your arms constantly in motion, staggered from one another. The ultimate goal is to have your nose safely touch the floor with each push-up for optimal range of motion. Performing one staggered push-up equates to one repetition.

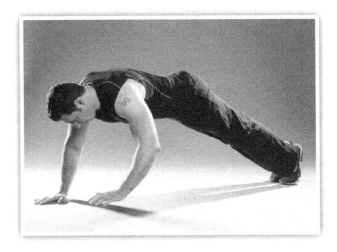

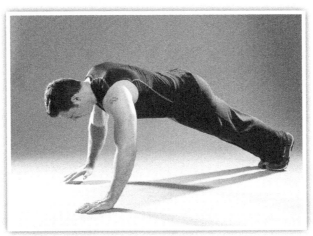

Beginner: Three sets total, 12 repetitions each
Intermediate: Three sets total, 16 repetitions each

Advanced: Four sets total, 20 repetitions each

Rest time between sets should be two to four minutes for recovery.

Tips: Do not lean, shift, or hike your hips during this push-up. Furthermore, be mindful to not dip your shoulder or elevate your upper trapezius for stability. Remember to place your hands down softly on the floor from one repetition to the next. You do not want to place your hands down too forcefully since this could cause potential injury to your wrists, elbows, or shoulders. If positioning your hands a little more than shoulder-width apart proves too challenging, you may position your hands out wider from your shoulders for added core stability. However, when that position is no longer challenging, attempt the push-up with the previous more challenging position. Be mindful to complete a full push-up and extend your elbows upward before moving into the next staggered moving hand placement. Remember "The Focused Five," particularly to keep your core in the neutral spinal position throughout.

4. Walk Out Push-ups

After mastering moving your hands in both staggered and in-to-out approaches, the next progression is to move your hands forward and backward. This exercise challenges the core stabilization and core movement muscles with optimal effectiveness by adjusting your hand placement to reach far past the shoulder-width position of a traditional push-up. Due to the range of motion provided in this push-up, there is no need to execute excessive height with your hand placement, nor will you drag your hands off the floor with each repetition. Your hands will be continuously moving forward and backward with great speed to provide the power in this exercise. Additionally, the farther you bring your hands forward, the more your latissimus dorsi muscles, hamstrings, and calves will become engaged, and therefore stretched in the process. This push-up builds lean muscle in the primary movers of this exercise, which are the anterior and medial deltoid muscles, pectoralis major and pectoralis minor muscles, triceps, gluteus maximus muscle, quadriceps, hamstrings, and calves. Your rhomboids and other back muscles are providing the proper stabilization to assist during this push-up. At this stage of your push-up journey, your core stabilization and core movement muscles are very strong. Thus, they will aide with the shoulder and triceps strength needed for optimal performance.

Starting Position: As with the other push-up beginning positions, keep your legs locked, with knees and feet together to properly engage your core and maintain a neutral spinal position in your back. Your heels should be slightly forward. Next, place your hands slightly more than shoulder-width apart.

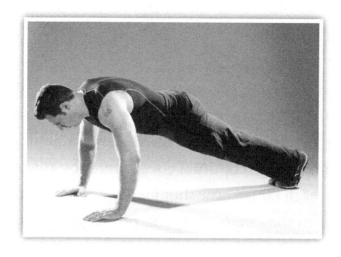

To Perform: Lower yourself downward with your nose gently touching the floor and then rise up back to the starting position with your knees, legs, and feet together. Next, continuously move both hands slightly forward (away from your shoulders) a few inches in between each push-up until your hands are far past your shoulders. To finalize a complete round, now reverse the sequence, moving your hands back towards the shoulders about two inches in between each push-up repetition until getting back to the starting position. For optimal effectiveness, attempt six repetitions forward and then six repetitions backward for one complete round. In general, maintain a consistent yet comfortable tempo while executing each push-up.

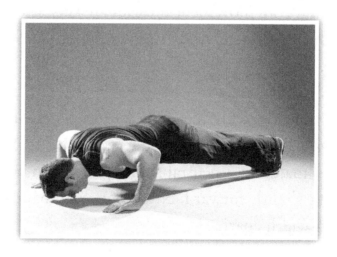

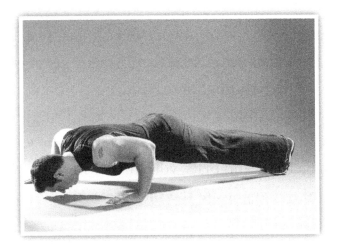

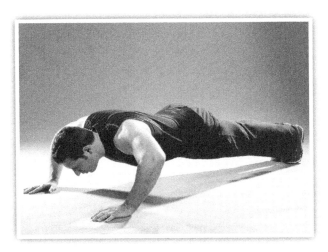

Beginners: Three sets total, one set is considered one round of performing six push-ups forward and then six push-ups backward. Intermediate: Three sets total, one set is considered two rounds of performing six push-ups forward and then six push-ups backward. Advanced: Three sets total, one set is considered three rounds of performing six push-ups forward and then six push-ups backward.

Rest time between sets should be two to four minutes for recovery.

Tips: It's crucial for the core to maintain a neutral spinal position during this movement since your hands are moving steadily forward and then backward. Do not be tempted to move your lower body while performing this push-up. Every muscle below the pelvis must remain stationary for optimal core recruitment keeping your knees, legs, and feet together throughout. Also, be cautious not to elevate your upper trapezius muscles for strength when bringing your hands forward. Remember to take very small steps with your hands for proper core engagement and place your hands softly on the floor with each repetition to not aggravate the shoulders, elbows, or wrists.

5. Kick Backs with Push-ups

This push-up is a classic power exercise since you will be bringing your legs backward while jumping. This exercise provides an incredible stretch to practically every muscle below your pelvis due to the power movement of jumping. Furthermore, this exercise provides the stability in your anterior and medial deltoids, latissimus dorsi muscles, middle trapezius, rhomboids, and triceps while the strength is provided in your pectoralis major and minor, and those shoulder muscles. What truly makes this exercise very challenging is that your knees, legs, and feet must stay together during the "kick back" portion of this exercise. It would be much easier if your knees and legs were not together with your feet positioned at shoulder-width apart. However, by keeping your knees, legs, and feet together you now have everything below the pelvis working as one unit which creates more core stabilization and engages more core movement muscles.

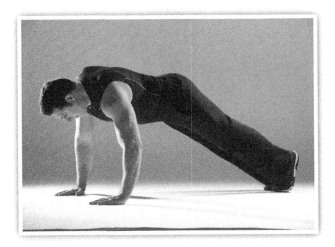

Starting Position: Begin with your chest facing the floor with your hands slightly more than shoulder-width apart. Your knees, legs, and feet are together to promote optimal core stability with your toes slightly forward.

To Perform: Lower yourself into a push-up with your nose gently touching the floor. To complete the push-up, rise up and keep your elbows slightly bent while you gently hop both of your knees, legs, and feet together toward your chest. Then bring your knees, legs, and feet together backward creating excessive height in the air. Your knees should start out flexed (bent), but then extend (lock) fully as your feet gently touch the floor back into the starting position to finish the exercise. One repetition equates to one push-up and one kick back. These push-ups should be executed with constant speed and height to obtain optimal power.

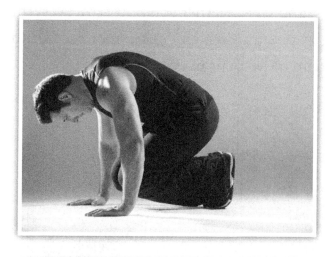

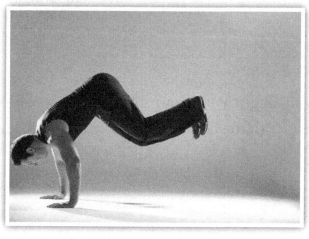

Beginner: Three sets total, five repetitions each
Intermediate: Three sets total, 10 repetitions each
Advanced: Three sets total, 15 repetitions each

Rest time between sets should be two to four minutes for recovery.

Tips: Range of motion is vital while performing this exercise. For example, your knees should touch the bottom of your chest and then be fully extended back into the starting position throughout upon each repetition. You may use your palms for added stability to assist in strength during this exercise. Remember to always keep your elbows slightly bent to keep tension on all of the core muscles and upper body muscles. If this exercise is too challenging to start, you may make this exercise easier by separating your legs (knees are no longer touching) and keeping your feet positioned at shoulder-width apart. However, keep the knees, legs, and feet together when able during the push-up portion for full core movement and stabilization muscle recruitment. Remember to maintain a neutral spinal position during this push-up and do not be tempted to round your back when attempting to have your knees touch your chest. Continue to apply the "Focused Five" during this push-up.

6. Mountain Climbers with Push-ups

This exercise challenges your lower and upper body for optimal core recruitment due to the duration of time it takes to complete a full set. Foremost, your upper body muscles are completely engaged throughout, both in movement and stabilization during this push-up. The time-under-tension that this push-up produces is phenomenal both for functional and aesthetic goals. Moreover, the mountain climber portion of this push-up can be considered as "horizontal running" while the power comes from the speed used when hopping throughout with each repetition. As with the power push-ups you have performed before, this "hopping" movement will provide an incredible stretch to every muscle below your pelvis. This exercise will also produce lean muscle in your gluteus maximus, hamstrings, quadriceps, and calves. Other primary movers in your upper body for this exercise are: anterior and medial deltoid muscles, pectoralis major and pectoralis minor muscles, and triceps. Your back muscles such as the rhomboids and middle trapezius are providing constant stabilization during this exercise.

Starting Position: Begin with your chest facing the floor with your hands slightly more than shoulder-width apart. Your knees, legs, and feet are together to promote optimal core stability.

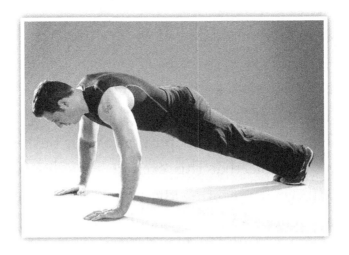

To Perform: Lower yourself into a push-up with your nose touching the floor. To complete the push-up, rise up and keep your elbows slightly bent while you bend one knee bringing it to your chest with a "hop" to your step. Your other foot remains stationary on the floor with your heel up. Then repeat the same action with your other leg creating another "hop" to your step as you bring your knee to your chest. Continue to alternate your legs with the most speed as possible. Performing one push-up and two fast moving mountain climbers with each leg equals one full repetition.

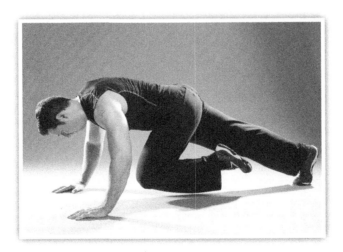

Beginner: Three sets total, 10 repetitions each
Intermediate: Four sets total, 12 repetitions each
Advanced: Four sets total, 16 repetitions each

Rest time between sets should be two to four minutes for recovery.

Tips: Remember to always keep your elbows bent to keep tension on the core and upper body muscles. Be especially quick when performing the mountain climber portion of this push-up to obtain the most power possible that this exercise provides. The range of motion is critical when executing the mountain climber portion of this movement. Hence, your knee should always touch the bottom of your chest throughout for each repetition. As always, maintain a neutral spinal position during this push-up and do not be tempted to round your back when attempting to have your knee touch your chest. Rounding your back only contributes to creating scapulae protraction. Again, this is particularly harmful since your scapulae muscles become over-active (tight), lose range of motion and strength, and contribute to muscular imbalances. Remember to engage all of your core stability and core movement muscles during this push-up. Don't forget to apply "The Focused Five!"

7. Crab Walk Push-ups

Your power push-up journey is almost complete and every push-up thus far has prepared for you for this exercise. It entails constant hand and leg movement while moving your entire body from side to side. This dynamic movement challenges your muscles intensely to work in an unusual way, creating a multitude of coordination while stretching your leg muscles and lower back. Furthermore, this exercise requires cardiovascular ability since your core, upper body, and lower body must work together for optimal strength since your hip flexors must maintain a neutral spinal position in your back throughout. The primary movers of this exercise that build lean muscle are: anterior, medial, and posterior deltoid muscles, pectoralis major and pectoralis minor muscles, triceps, rhomboids, latissimus dorsi muscles, rotator cuffs, hip flexors, hip adductors, erector spinae, gluteus maximus muscles, gluteus minimus muscles, gluteus medius muscles, hamstrings, and calves.

Starting Position: As with most of the beginning push-up positions above, start in the traditional push-up position with your knees, feet, and legs together. Your hands should be positioned slightly more than shoulder-width apart.

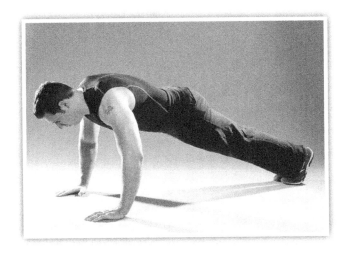

To Perform: Execute a push-up with your nose touching the floor for optimal range of motion and then shuffle with intense speed horizontally to one side. Shuffle simultaneously with your hands and feet to one side, and then perform a push-up with your knees, legs, and feet together throughout. Next, shuffle back to your starting position and perform another push-up with your knees, legs, and feet together. The number of shuffles you perform side-to-side and the volume of push-ups depend obviously on your fitness levels (please see detailed information below). To finish a set, alternate from side-to-side and perform a push-up after you execute your shuffles.

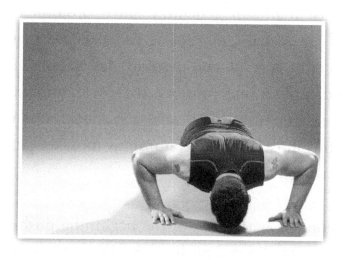

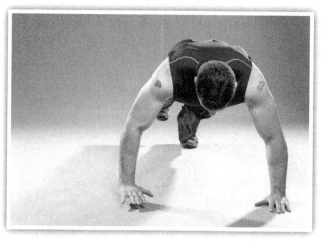

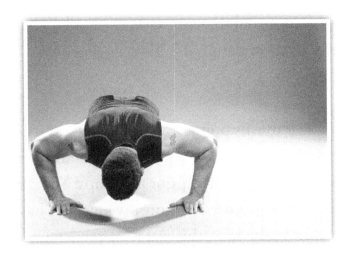

Beginner: Three sets total, 12 repetitions, six repetitions each side, two shuffles

Intermediate: Three sets total, 20 repetitions, 10 repetitions each side, three shuffles

Advanced: Three sets total, 30 repetitions, 15 repetitions each side, four shuffles

Rest time between sets should be three to four minutes for full recovery.

Tips: Remember to maintain a neutral spinal position throughout. Be incredibly cautious not to have your lower back form an inward curve, causing your hips to drop excessively. Similarly, do not round your back, which raises your gluteus maximus muscles higher than your hips. Both of these incorrect methods can cause stress to your lower back without developing functional core strength in the stabilization and movement muscles. If this exercise becomes too strenuous, you may pause and then continue when able. Be mindful to not cross your arms or you feet during this movement, especially if you become fatigued. Crossing will prevent the core from achieving its proper stabilization and movement function while the rotator cuff will not benefit from optimal stabilization either. Finally, challenge yourself to execute these push-ups applying "The Focused Five" to their fullest capacity throughout.

If you have made it to this point of your push-up journey, you deserve a huge congratulations and an incredible amount of validation for being able to complete all of the prior push-ups! Your consistency and dedication are nothing short of impressive, as you have had to work extremely hard to make it to this point of your journey. You should see real aesthetic changes in your body from all of these push-ups you have previously performed. Your upper and lower body should have more lean muscle with decreased body fat. Furthermore, your core should also aesthetically look equally as impressive. Most importantly, functional stabilization and movement in your body should be very much improved including your posture. Your stability, strength, and power ability should all be incredibly developed. Again, your motivation has driven you to this final push-up. Nice work!

8. Jumping Jack Push-ups

The final push-up in your journey will be a challenging one since it combines all of the prior teachings of stability, strength, and power in one exercise. Your shoulders, chest, back muscles, and core stabilization muscles all provide optimal stabilization in the beginning of this push-up and during the act of performing the jumping jack. Next, the action of physically performing this push-up builds strength in your shoulders, chest, triceps, and core movement muscles. Possessing unsurpassed leg power is required to perform the jumping jack portion of this push-up along with creating great height. This exercise builds lean muscle in your anterior and medial shoulders, pectoralis major and minor muscles, triceps, and every muscle below your pelvis including all of your gluteal muscles. Additionally, because of the range of motion in your legs provided by this push-up movement, this exercise provides an incredible stretch to your hips along with engaging your hip adductors and hip abductors muscles.

Starting Position: As with most of the beginning push-up positions above, start in the traditional push-up position with your knees, feet, and legs together with your toes slightly rotated forward. Your hands should be positioned slightly more than shoulder-width apart.

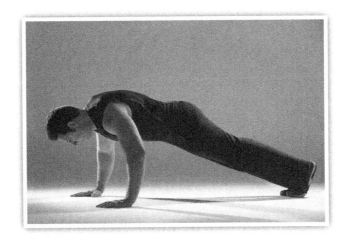

To Perform: Execute a push-up with your nose safely touching the floor for optimal range of motion and then as you rise back up to the starting position, jump out your legs (in a "V" shape) as wide as possible with as much height as you are able to obtain. While performing the jumping jacks, be sure to extend (lock) your knees for optimal posterior chain recruitment in your hamstrings and calves. Then after performing the jumping jack in the air, land softly back into the starting position. Keep repeating creating extreme speed and height during your jumping jacks to obtain the optimal power in this push-up. One jumping jack and one push-up equates to one repetition.

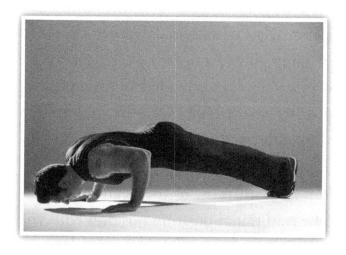

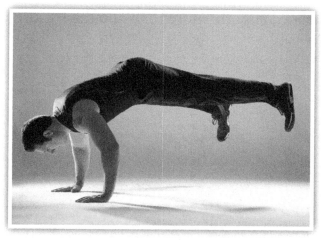

Beginner: Three sets total, 10 repetitions each

Intermediate: Three sets total, 16 repetitions each
Advanced: Three sets total, 24 repetitions each

Rest time between sets should be two to four minutes for full recovery.

Tips: Do not hesitate executing the jumping jack portion of this exercise after performing the push-up. Performing any hesitation doesn't provide the proper speed or force required to make this a power push-up. Moreover, some unnecessary reluctance could cause strain to your shoulders and wrists that might result in possible injury. You may use force in your upper body including your palms for stabilization to assist in creating the excessive height that this push-up demands. Remember to maintain a neutral spinal position during every portion of this push-up. As always, be cautious not to have your lower back create an inward curve, which results in your hips to drop excessively. Correspondingly, do not round your back, which raises your gluteus maximus muscles higher than your hips and creates scapulae protraction. Both of these incorrect methods can cause stress to your lower back without developing core power in the stabilization and movement muscles. If this exercise becomes too strenuous or too challenging, you may execute the jumping jack portion of this push-up with less height and speed. Remember you may always pause and then continue when able while executing this exercise. Apply "The Focused Five" for optimal assistance during this push-up.

PART V

Common Muscular Imbalances & Corrections

Upper Extremity Disorder

This postural disorder can be easy to diagnose since it can best be defined as having protracted shoulders (shoulders that fall forward). The over-active (tight) muscles associated with Upper Extremity Disorder (UED) are: pectoralis major, pectoralis minor, anterior deltoids, and the latissimus dorsi. The muscles that are under-active (weak) are rhomboids, middle and lower trapezius.

UED can develop in the body for multiple reasons. First, if you are an individual that happens to sit extensively during the day or has an occupation that requires you to type on a computer for prolonged periods of time, UED can occur quickly. This is due to the act of flexion in your over-active muscles that sitting provides. These muscles are your latissimus dorsi, hip flexors, hamstrings, anterior shoulders, and your pectoralis muscles. Moreover, excessive sitting doesn't engage your under-active muscles and contributes to more muscular imbalances such as improper posture.

Second, if you are someone who trains your anterior deltoids, pectoralis muscles, and latissimus dorsi muscles regularly without incorporating proper stretching techniques to these specific muscles groups, then the muscle fibers shorten and become tighter. When this muscular imbalance begins to occur, then UED starts to occur in your body.

Third, you train these over-active muscles without working the muscles that are under-active. As such, you must create some kind of strength training program to have these under-active muscles become stronger to support all of the training that the over-active muscles obtain either in your functional daily life or during exercise.

Those who have UED can still benefit from performing push-ups since you wouldn't want those over-active muscles to atrophy. Although, as stated, it is crucial to properly stretch the over-active muscles while strengthening the under-active muscles. For example, execute the wall stretch or prisoner stretch (in the Stretching Section) to stretch your pectoralis major, pectoralis minor, and anterior deltoids. The overhead stretch (also located in the upcoming Stretching Section) is a beneficial stretch to your latissimus dorsi muscles. Furthermore, applying self-myofacial release by stretching your latissimus dorsi with the foam roller can be extremely effective, holding the pose for 20 to 30 seconds. Remember to stretch your dominant side one to two more times to encourage symmetry in the body.

While the push-ups in this book engage all of the over-active muscles that contribute to having UED, there are some push-ups in this book that strengthen the scapulae and rhomboids to help correct UED. Nevertheless, to best strengthen these weak muscles such as the rhomboids specifically, attempt the pronated dumbbell row. You can stabilize yourself with a weight bench or against the weight rack while you row underneath your chest holding the dumbbell with your palms down keeping a slight arch to your back (legs and feet are together, knees flexed). Your upper back should remain relaxed and not rounded during the rowing exercise. Perform the pronated row with a weight you can comfortably lift for three sets with eight repetitions to build proper strength and hypertrophy to these muscles.

Another great strength training exercise to perform to help correct UED is scaption. Scaption builds lean muscle in your scapulae and rhomboids that will functionally strengthen your rotator cuff, specifically the supraspinatus, all while encouraging optimal posture to your body. Scaption also creates shoulder mobility that will fortify your joints and tendons. By performing scaption, over time, you will become stronger in other pressing or lateral movements such as performing push-ups. To perform, stand with your feet shoulder-width apart with optimal posture and hold a dumbbell in each hand with your palms facing you in a neutral grip position. Next, bring both dumbbells up into a "Y" formation at a 45-degree angle. Be cautious to not raise the dumbbell higher than your shoulders, since this would engage the upper trapezius (which is counter-productive to this particular exercise). Remember to engage your core and gluteus muscles to help build strength and maintain optimal posture when executing this exercise. Perform three sets of eight to 12 repetitions.

Anterior Pelvic Tilt

This muscular imbalance is one of the most common in our current general population. It can best be defined as when the pelvis tilts forward extremely. It can be easy to spot in the mirror if you turn to your side when looking at yourself. You do not want to have an excessive arch in your lower back while standing. This arching occurs from a combination of over-active and under-active muscles. First, the over-active (tight) muscles are the hip flexors (iliacus and psoas muscles) and erector spinae. Your hip flexors provide flexion to your hips, provide flexion to your abdominals and knees, assist in the movement of your legs in the transverse (horizontal plane) and in the frontal plane of motion, and support in stabilization for every muscle below your pelvis. As stated, your erector spinae is not actually just a singular muscle, but it's actually a collection of a variety of muscles and tendons that run vertically up your spine from your pelvis to your head. This assembly of muscles that make up your erector spinae aids in bending and twisting your spine in a variety of directions along with providing spinal stability while standing. As a result, your hip flexors and erector spinae provide a multitude of useful functional benefits for your body. Excessive sitting daily at work or home only causes your hip-flexors and erector spinae to become more over-active. Therefore, do your best to stand-up and walk around even for only a few minutes every one to two hours when sitting for long periods. This act of moving around will prevent your hip flexors and erector spinae from tightening up and creating more of an anterior tilt in your body. Definitely keep in mind that inefficient movements, either in your daily functional life or while strength training, can strain and tighten your erector spinae muscles as well.

There are numerous forms of stretching you can perform to lengthen these over-active muscles. For instance, stretch the hip flexor muscles and erector spinae by utilizing the foam roller. As noted, the foam roller is a great tool to provide release to these muscles, holding each stretch for 30 seconds. Again, you will want to stretch your dominant side one to two times more than the less under-active side. You may perform static stretches for your hip flexors such as the kneeling hip flexor stretch, pigeon pose stretch, and hip crossover stretch. Active stretches providing movement can be very beneficial to stretch your hip flexors, too. Those stretches are: leg swings, rear lunges, lying marching, and Romanian lunges. Some great static stretches for your erector spinae that lengthen your spine and create extension are the cat pose, kneeling stability ball latissimus dorsi stretch, lateral flexion stretch, and standing back-bend stretch.

The under-active (weak) muscles are the gluteal muscles, which are your gluteus maximus, gluteus medius, and gluteus minimus. To strengthen the gluteal muscles, you may perform any of the stability push-up exercises in this book because these are the principle exercises to maintain the neutral spinal position. If your pelvic tilt is just creating too much trouble for you to maintain the neutral spinal position, then perform stationary lunges, step-ups on a minimum of a foot incline, and floor bridges to strengthen your gluteus maximus muscles. Performing three sets of eight to 12 repetitions is best for strength. Next, the gluteus medius muscle is the primary hip abductor that creates movement away from your body, thus providing a stretch to your hip flexors and enabling the anterior pelvic tilt. Performing the Jumping Jack Push-ups, Alternating Side Extension Push-ups, Isometric Side Leg Extension Push-ups, and Isometric T-Rotation Push-ups all engage the gluteus medius muscles. Other exercises that provide strength to your gluteus medius muscles are side planks and lying side leg extensions. These exercises should also be executed for eight to 12 repetitions for three sets. Finally, the gluteus minimus can be considered part of your hips because they also help bring your legs laterally out to the side, much like your gluteus medius muscles. Performing the Jumping Jack Push-ups, Alternating Side Extension Push-ups, Isometric Side Leg Extension Push-ups, and Isometric T-Rotation Push-ups all also engage your gluteus medius muscles. Side planks and clams are also effective exercises to engage these gluteal muscles for three sets of eight to 12 repetitions.

You may still perform push-ups with an anterior pelvic tilt, however, it may prove difficult to maintain and perform the neutral spinal position. For that reason, it's still critical to strengthen and stretch those specific muscles to prevent your pelvis from tilting forward. By correcting an anterior pelvic tilt, you encourage ideal posture and achieve the optimal core stabilization and core movement muscles for complete activation. Furthermore, by correcting your anterior pelvic tilt, or even minimizing this postural distortion, you prevent inefficient movements patterns, which often leads to potential injury.

Stretches

Stretching is crucial to perform since you need to create equal symmetry in your muscles by lengthening them after exercise. Strength training via performing a variety of push-ups can tighten a muscle and make those specific muscles over-active. Engaging a muscle always equates to shortening it, which is great because that's the recruitment we want to build muscle. However, shortening a muscle too much without also lengthening it could result into loss of range of motion and possible injury. Enclosed below are four helpful static stretches to help you balance your muscles correctly.

1. Wall Stretch

This is a fantastic stretch to perform for your pectoralis major, pectoralis minor, anterior shoulders, and medial shoulders. Again, your chest and shoulder muscles are the primary movers engaged during push-ups. You will want to perform this stretch after your push-up workout because this stretch is a static stretch. Do not perform this stretch *before* your workout since it would lengthen the muscle too much and could possibly lead to injury. You'll want to stretch both sides, however, stretch your more over-active (tighter) side one to two times more to create equal symmetry in the body. If you always stretch both your left and right sides to the same degree, then you will always have one side that is more over-active.

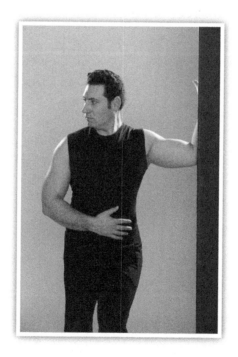

To perform: If you are stretching your left side first, then position your left forearm with a neutral grip (palm facing yourself) on the doorframe or corner of the wall. Your right hand should be wrapped around your torso or on your stomach. Your left foot will be positioned about two feet from your torso. Bend your left knee forward while your right foot is behind your gluteal muscles with a slight bend to your knee. Next, turn to your right side while holding this stretch for 30 seconds. You can make this stretch more intense by how much you bend your front knee forward and how much you fully turn your torso to the opposite side. Remember to stretch your more over-active side three to four times, and then your other side two times total to create equal symmetry in your body.

2. Triceps Stretch

This is a great stretch to engage the triceps after you have performed your push-ups. Your triceps are much smaller muscles than your chest and shoulder muscles, however, they are crucial to stretch since your triceps become the secondary movers during your push-ups. Remember because this stretch is a static stretch, you'll want to perform it after your workout because you don't want to lengthen a muscle too much since this could create possible injury. Again, you'll want to stretch both sides, however, stretch your more over-active (tighter) side one to two times more to create symmetry in the body.

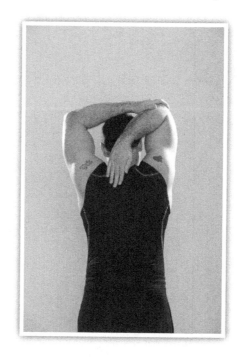

To perform: Stand with optimal posture with your feet positioned shoulder-width apart. If you're stretching your right side first, raise your right arm and bend it backward with your right hand on your upper trapezius muscle, elbow pointing up. Your left hand is placed on your right elbow as you push downward gently, creating the tension to stretch the right triceps. You could make this stretch more intense by how much pressure you place with your left hand on your right elbow. Hold this stretch for 30 seconds and perform on both sides, however, perform more repetitions on the over-active side to create the symmetry that we have gone over in this section.

3. Overhead Stretch

This is a wonderful stretch to perform for your latissimus dorsi, pectoralis major and minor muscles, anterior deltoids, triceps, and forearms. The latissimus dorsi muscles are vital to stretch because they are part of your core movement muscles, and a stabilizer muscle in a variety of the push-ups that you have performed. This stretch is also considered a static stretch and should be performed after your push-up workout.

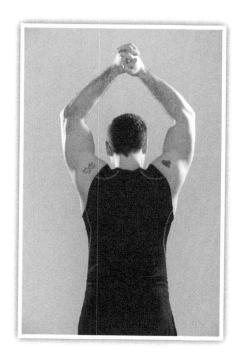

To perform: Start with positioning your feet shoulder-width apart and stand with optimal posture. Bring both of your hands in front of your waist and intertwine both of your hands together. Next, clasp your hands together and raise them above your head with locked (straight) elbows. Do your best to bring both of your arms over your head past ear-level without hyperextending your lower back. You may have a slight arch to your lower back. If you have an anterior pelvic tilt, however, be sure that you are not creating an excessive arch to bring both of your arms back further. Be sure to perform three to four sets and hold for 30 seconds after your push-up workout.

4. Prisoner Stretch

This is a wonderful stretch for your pectoralis major and minor muscles, anterior deltoids, triceps, and forearms. Again, your chest and shoulder muscles are the primary movers engaged during push-ups. This stretch is also considered a static stretch and should be performed after your push-up workout.

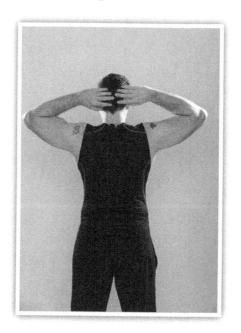

To perform: Stand with optimal posture with your feet positioned at shoulder-width apart with both of your hands positioned behind the back of your head. Be sure to have both of your left and right fingers intertwined to create a shorter range of motion for your hand positioning. This will result in a more concentrated stretch for your muscles. Once you have your hand positioning correct, move your elbows backward while squeezing your scapulae (shoulder-blades) together. You can make this stretch more intense depending on how much force you create by bringing your arms backward. To get the best results from this stretch, perform three to four sets and hold for 30 seconds after your push-up workout.

SAFETY DISCLAIMER

Foremost, you know your body better than anyone. It's vital to listen to your body before, during, and after exercising. Please do not hesitate to consult your primary doctor or a sports medicine physician if you feel any kind of pain while performing the exercises in this book. Pain is never a good occurrence while exercising and it's your body's method of letting you know that something could be wrong. If you have a history of high blood pressure, hypertension, heart disease, or any other extreme disease, please again consult your physician before exercising to confirm that you are healthy enough to perform this program. Additionally, if you experience any sharp or intense pain in your shoulders, lower back, wrists, or anywhere else while attempting these push-ups, please stop and contact your physician.

CONCLUSION

Be proud of yourself for picking up and reading this book! Then be extremely proud of yourself for completing the 24 push-up journey! You made a powerful choice by choosing to take this journey and investing in yourself. Fitness is always a choice and you chose to be healthy. If you've made it this far, you've obtained a multitude of knowledge in regards to the core, the push-up, and all of their benefits. After completing your own push-up journey, you will have acquired more functional core strength, more lean muscle throughout your body, stronger stability in your joints, overall power, and proper posture. Moreover, and most importantly, you will also be much healthier! I admire your commitment and dedication to transforming your body by taking this journey with me. By now you can fully appreciate how the push-up can be a tremendous cardiovascular workout, along with anaerobically working the upper body, lower body, and core stabilization and movement muscles. I realize that many of these push-ups may have been challenging and that this may not have been the easiest of journeys. Remember, though, that not all accomplishments easily change you both physically *and* mentally. Also bear in mind that no matter your overall fitness performance level, you can always progress these push-ups further by performing more sets, more repetitions, or taking shorter rest periods. You may have completed this 24 push-up journey, but it doesn't have to end here. Let this book be the beginning of your own lifelong journey, and now apply your favorite or most challenging push-ups into your other fitness routines. You now have the "core" of a lifetime of fitness. Therefore, let it be your guide to a healthier and stronger you!

I wish you continued success and the best of health through this push-up journey and beyond.

ABOUT THE AUTHOR

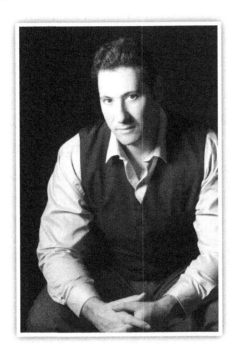

As the son of a professional bodybuilder, Shaun was exposed to weightlifting and exercise at a very young age. After overcoming his own physical limitations, having been born with club feet and gross motor skills, Shaun made it his mission to share his passion and knowledge of proper fitness and health to help others meet their fitness goals.

For over ten years, Shaun has successfully run his own personal training business in the New York City Metro area. Able to relate and adapt to each individual, Shaun prides himself on developing exercise plans and nutritional menus to foster every client's fitness needs. His clientele ranges from the athlete and senior citizen to the bodybuilder and dancer. Shaun's specialties include strength training, power techniques, corrective injury training, and core stability training.

In addition to the highly regarded Master Trainer status, Shaun is a certified personal trainer of the National Academy of Sports Medicine (NASM). With NASM Shaun also holds specialized certifications in Pre- and Post-Natal, Corrective Exercise Practices, Cardiovascular Weight Loss, Youth Training, Senior Citizen Training, Balance Training, Core Stabilization, and Self Myofascial Release (SMR). Additionally, Shaun is certified by the International Sports Science Association (ISSA) as a Sports Performance Nutrition Specialist, with training in the Female Athlete, Knee & Shoulder Rehabilitation, and Marathon Training. Shaun earned his Bachelor's degree in English Literature and Writing from the University of Delaware.

Shaun's first full-length book, the first edition of "Push-up Progression," was featured as one of three top books in 2013 for healthy living as selected by Dr. John Whyte of The Discovery Channel. Shaun has had a multitude of articles, program designs, and tips published within a variety of books, magazines, and on websites in the world of fitness and beyond, including: Price World Publishing, Demos Medical Publishing, Livestrong, Rodale Books, OnFitness Magazine, Fitness Magazine, Brides Magazine, and GO: AirTran Magazine. Additionally, Fitness Professional Online recognizes Shaun as an "expert," answering questions for other fitness and health professionals.

Shaun also has media experience in both television and radio, ranging from fitness modeling to hosting his own weekly radio fitness show.

For more information about Shaun Zetlin, visit:
http://www.zetlinfitness.com/

Made in the USA
Middletown, DE
26 September 2023